A Personal Note

Thank you for enroling in CHIP! You have made a wise decision—probably one of your best decisions ever—in signing up for the Complete Health Improvement Program! You are joining more than 50,000 CHIP graduates who have experienced remarkable and measurable improvements in their health. Many of these results have been published in peer-reviewed medical journals and have caught the attention of public health experts around the world.

CHIP does this by encouraging a greater measure of self-care in the context of good medical care. Through intensive group education in a supportive environment, CHIP focuses on bringing a clearer understanding of the nature and causes of today's chronic diseases, their risk factors, and how to prevent, treat, disarm and potentially reverse them. How? By helping you adopt a lifestyle with proven results and priceless benefits.

As well as getting you hooked on a more active lifestyle, we'll expose you to a better way of eating. You will learn how to widen your use of delicious whole foods, such as fruits and vegetables, whole grains, beans and lentils, and some nuts. These foods are high in nutrients, fiber and satiety, yet low in calories, sugar, salt, fat and cholesterol. These foods don't need nutrition labels because they are nutritionally balanced naturally.

Yet CHIP does not follow dietary dogma. While what we call the Optimal Diet serves as a dietary goal, you can choose your level of implementation based on your motivation, clinical status and goals.

As you begin to better understand the cause-and-effect relationship between your lifestyle choices and health (or disease), we hope you will no longer choose the "good life" and its dietary excesses, choosing instead the "best life" possible, with its elegant simplicity and your new-found zest for living.

I always say that health may not be everything but without health, everything is nothing! So give this your best efforts.

With best wishes for health and happiness,

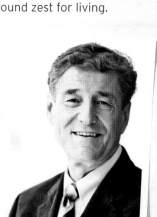

Hans Diehl

Hans A Diehl, DrHSc, MPH, FACN
CHIP Founder

Foreword

Over the past century, we've seen a dramatic change in the types of diseases we fear—and that we spend our money trying to fight. Chronic diseases such as obesity, diabetes, high cholesterol and high blood pressure threaten to make the current generation the first since statistics have been recorded to die at an average younger age than their parents. These chronic diseases are predominantly lifestyle diseases—fundamentally caused by lifestyle choices we make.

So if we're getting sicker and sicker with lifestyle-related diseases, it would make sense to approach this chronic disease epidemic with lifestyle-related treatments. That's what CHIP—the Complete Health Improvement Program—is: a proven lifestyle-related approach to disease prevention, treatment and reversal. If you read this book, and especially if you incorporate your reading of it into the full program, including the presentation, workbook, recipe book and other tools, you will be participating in the best and most complete scientifically validated community-based lifestyle medicine treatment program that exists!

Lifestyle-related diseases occur partly because of choices we make as individuals, and partly because of collective choices we have made as a society. Modern developments such as food processing, storage and transportation techniques, and automobiles, television and computers that have generally improved our lives have also brought with them unintended consequences. We didn't acquire these problems overnight and we won't change them overnight either. But if you, and the person next to you, and your doctor, your hospital, and your whole health care system incorporate the CHIP insights into your lives, we can change not only who we are as individuals, but also where our society is going.

This book can be used by individuals, families, communities and corporations to move our health in the right direction. CHIP is meant to change your life. Sometimes that's fun and easy. Sometimes it's frustrating and difficult. But if you stick with it, not only can you be a different person, you will also be helping make your area of the world a different place. So, have courage—enjoy each moment and know that you're doing great things, not only for yourself but also for others!

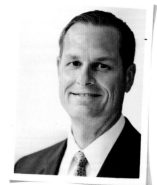

Wayne Dysinger, MD, MPH
Loma Linda University
American College of Lifestyle Medicine

Learn more

Lifestyle Medicine

While modern medicine has made great progress in the fight against infectious diseases and amazing technological advances, many chronic diseases are increasingly common. The predominant cause is lifestyle. Lifestyle medicine is an increasingly important—and increasingly researched—response to the growing incidence of lifestyle diseases. The lifestyle choices we make each day have the potential to significantly reduce our risks of—and potentially reverse—many diseases and help us on the path to optimal health.

Chapter One introduces the nature of medicine and healing, before demonstrating the startling rise of lifestyle disease. This is our first step toward changing how we see health and wellbeing.

Chapter Two provides an overview of the major research studies that have been conducted over recent decades in the field of lifestyle medicine. Around the world and across people groups, these studies have demonstrated the lifestyle factors that can reduce the risks of chronic disease and potentially lead to the reversal of certain chronic diseases.

Chapter Three discovers the most deadly and damaging of lifestyle diseases, and introduces the lifestyle prescription for optimal health.

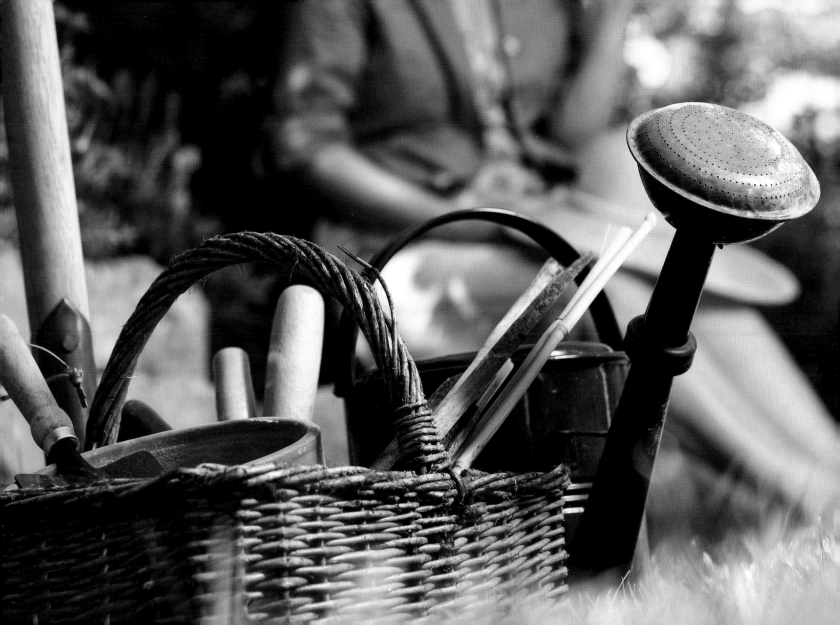

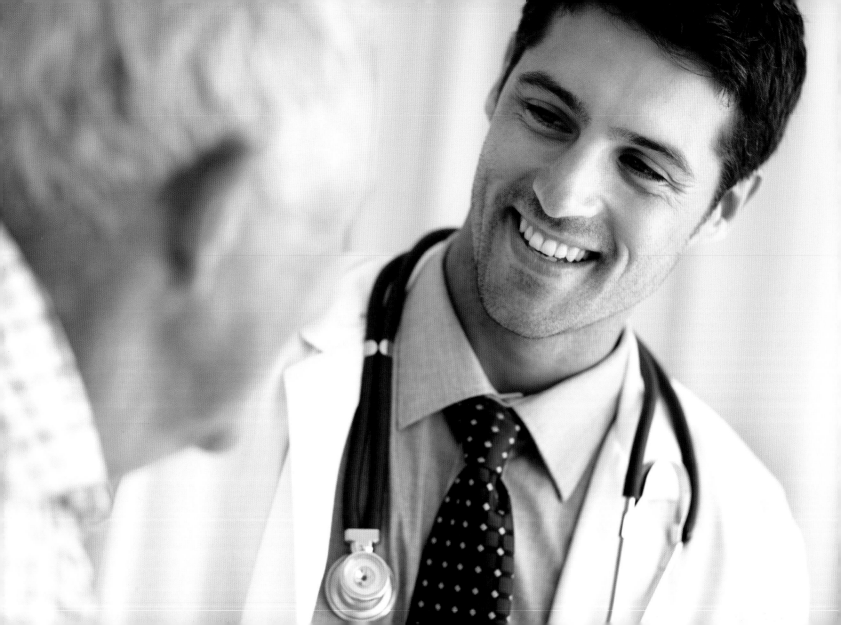

Chapter One

A Short History of Medicine and Healthcare

Faced with the choice, would you rather an illness you had be "controlled" with medications and procedures or have the potential to be reversed through changes in lifestyle behavior? The answer to this question lies at the heart of lifestyle medicine–a whole-person approach to health care that delves into finding and removing the causes–and therefore holds the key to both disease prevention and potential disease reversal. The exciting news is that today, you can choose to be healthy and live a potentially longer and fuller life. This choice is a feature of lifestyle medicine; a choice for optimal health and wellbeing. Through the journey and choices described in this book, you will have the tools you need to live your best and healthiest life.

In our modern world, despite many advances in medicine, we are seeing a frightening increase in a range of diseases and illnesses that are directly related to our modern way of living. In developed countries, an estimated 70 per cent of all visits to a doctor are thought to have a predominantly lifestyle-based cause.[1] Modernization itself can be seen as a major contributor to a range of chronic diseases, one that has an unmistakable connection to dietary and lifestyle factors. Many risk factors for these diseases and conditions are under our control. While other factors such as our genetic makeup and culture do have an impact, we can actively manage many elements of lifestyle in order to sustain or improve health. Factors that contribute to illness can be potentially turned around to contribute to wellness.

An estimated 70 per cent of all visits to a doctor are thought to have a predominantly lifestyle-based cause.

The historical view of medicine

Modern medicine has progressed in ways previous generations could not have imagined. Many medical procedures of old now seem odd to us: for example, we no longer let blood for infections or prescribe poisonous arsenic for common ailments. Without proper hygiene and limited medicines, hospitals were often places where the spread of disease and death were more common than healing.

Medicine has become a highly developed industry and the advances of recent decades have been described as the "pharmacological revolution." We have a vast range of pharmaceutical drugs that have been developed with years of testing and can save lives. Medical practitioners have typically been some of the great students and thinkers of their time, and advances in technology and research have allowed many acute and life-threatening illnesses to be controlled or reduced to the point they are almost non-existent—infectious diseases, such as polio and diphtheria, are good examples.

Vaccinations for these and many other infectious diseases, such as smallpox and measles, have helped reduce infant mortality rates and improve the health of populations in less-developed countries. The discovery of penicillin, an antibiotic derived from mold or fungi by Alexander Fleming in 1928, has long been considered a remarkable milestone in health care. Antibiotics are a fast and effective treatment for many infectious diseases.

Many accidents or illnesses—that would have been life threatening in the past—can now be healed and lead to a full recovery with the techniques of surgery and medicines developed in the past century. Medicine's ability to diagnose or test for the presence of disease or disturbances in the body has been supported by dramatic advances in laboratory techniques and treatment procedures that can target the precise causes of illness, with great confidence. X-ray, MRI and CAT scan technologies have allowed us to peer into the workings of the body without a need to open the skin, and we have a much deeper understanding of the complex workings of the systems within the body as a result. Anesthetics, which allow both local or general sensation and consciousness control, have been vital in all types of surgeries and treatments, allowing procedures to be given to a patient that would otherwise be impossible.

Our general standards of health care and medicine have also improved in the past century with the development of hygiene practices that change how disease is passed on. Clean water supplies, proper sanitation practices and nutritional advice have been important tools that have provided many improvements to living standards and health.

In 1862, Louis Pasteur refined a technique called "pasteurization" that changed how we managed food spoilage and bacteria-related illness from foods and liquids, especially milk. Sterilization and other developments such as antiseptics also supported infectious disease control in communities, and in surgeries and hospitals. There is little doubt that our ability to respond to acute and life-threatening illness with modern medicine is remarkable.

WHAT IS MEDICINE?

The main model of medicine today is called allopathic medicine, a term that refers to "a method of treating disease by the use of agents producing effects different from those of the disease treated" (The Macquarie Dictionary). This means that an illness will be responded to with a drug or treatment that is different to the symptom, in an attempt to change the symptom. This may set up a "symptom-medication" reaction that might not fully seek out the underlying cause of illness, nor encourage a preventive approach. Allopathic medicine is also called traditional or conventional medicine, and, for example, can include the typical experience of visiting a doctor and being written a prescription for a pharmaceutical product or treatment. While this plays an important role in managing disease, there are additional health care options that can further contribute to optimal health and wellbeing.

WHAT IS HEALTH CARE?

Health care is a broader concept and more in line with the philosophy of lifestyle medicine. The Medical Dictionary defines health care as "the prevention, treatment and management of illness and the preservation of mental and physical wellbeing through the services offered by the medical and allied health professions." This understanding can also be expanded to include how we create healthy environments and communities through adequate hygiene (clean water, proper sanitation), clean air, access to fresh produce, suitable shelter, and minimal pollutants and toxins.

What has changed?

Medicine's ability to treat acute and infectious disease is one of the great achievements of modern human history. So why aren't we healthier? Instead, we are now seeing a dramatic increase in diseases that are chronic and lifestyle-related.

For example, according to a textbook published in 1928, "You can expect one heart attack per year in an average hospital in an average sized town."[2] But now, an average of 4000 heart attacks occur per day in the United States.[3] An estimated 33 per cent of all US deaths are due to cardiovascular disease and 25 per cent of deaths are due to cancer, amounting to almost 60 per cent of total deaths.

On one hand, advances in technology have brought improvements to our lives, especially in medical technology and the production of food. On the other hand, we have become an increasingly sedentary population where even the simple act of walking has often been replaced by car travel, and we no longer gather or grow our own food in order to have a meal. Fast food and highly processed foods in our local supermarkets have become so "normal" that our concept of what real food is has changed—at the expense of our fresh fruit and vegetable intake. Even though we have been promised solutions in the form of low-fat foods and special dietary products, obesity rates continue to rise and, with them, chronic disease rates also. In nations such as Japan where diets are increasingly "Westernized," the incidence of cardiovascular disease is now increasing alongside the expanding waistlines that have become all too common in Western society.

Advances in technology have brought improvements to our lives, especially in medical technology and the production of food.

Diabetes Trends (per cent of people with diabetes from 1935 to 2010 by age)

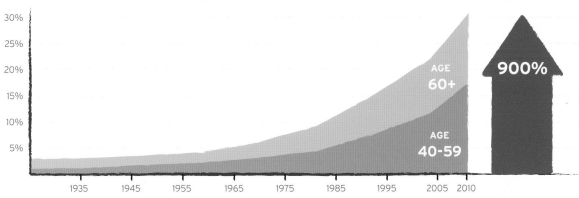

Obesity rates are rising so rapidly, it is now a global epidemic, along with many other chronic illnesses such as type 2 diabetes, heart disease, cancers and high blood pressure. One disturbing example is the increase in diabetes in many populations around the world. Despite stunning advances in medical knowledge and treatments during this time, diabetes rates in some age groups have increased by as much as 900 per cent since World War II, with the rates doubling every 20 years. Today, the risk of a newborn in the United States developing diabetes during their lifetime is one in three.[8] The US National Institutes of Health say we have no medical cure.

Obesity has serious implications for how we live and on our health, but it also affects those around us. As our waistlines expand, so do clothing sizes, furniture, door frames, and—on a more somber note—even casket sizes, cremation ovens and burial plots. Obesity also has far-reaching effects on the family, with the children of obese parents significantly more likely to be obese or to become obese adults. Younger generations are gaining weight at a faster rate than previous generations.

It sounds alarming but the answer to many of

Today, the risk of a newborn in the United States developing diabetes during their lifetime is one in three.

today's chronic diseases has been known for thousands of years. Around 400 BC, Hippocrates—considered the father of medicine—said that to keep well one should "avoid too much food, too little toil." We might now say "physical activity" instead of "toil" but the message is even more relevant today, more than 2400 years later.

IS THE RISE IN CHRONIC DISEASES SIMPLY DUE TO A LONGER LIFE SPAN TODAY?

Not as much as we might think. When we compare the average life expectancy of a baby born in developed nations in 1900 with that of today, we notice a difference of about 30 years, which might suggest that the medical model is working. However, this assumption is called into question when we notice that chronic diseases are happening in younger and younger people. In addition, infant mortality has been reduced significantly, which goes a considerable way toward explaining the 30-year difference in life expectancy at birth.

When we compare the life expectancy of an adult, we see a different picture. In 1900, for example, a 65 year old could expect to live to 77 years. Today, a 65 year old can expect to live to 85 years, offering an improvement of only about eight years.

And remember, that 77-year life expectancy in 1900 was accomplished with medicine still in its infancy. Today, 18 per cent of the United States' gross domestic income is given to medical care, of which 75 per cent is devoted to chronic diseases.[9]

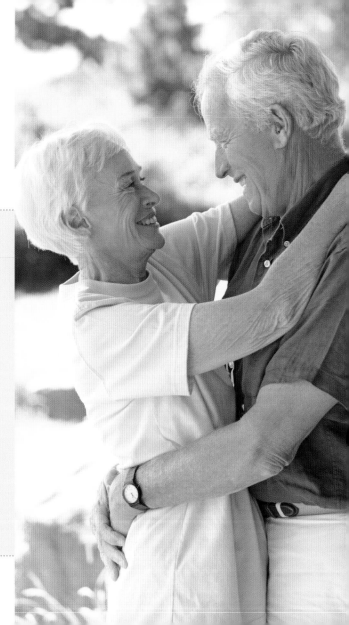

Responding to common diseases

Not only is Hippocrates's ancient wisdom still true, it is also being re-discovered and reconfirmed by medical and health researchers around the world. Researcher Dr Denis Burkitt put it like this: "The greatest discovery of the last 20 years was the understanding that our modern killer diseases are largely lifestyle related and therefore they must be preventable and potentially reversible."[10]

› Aging

Chronic disease and illness are not a natural part of the aging process despite the statistics that tell us disease rates are on the rise. In his book *The Blue Zones,* which looks closely at the lifestyle factors that have contributed to increased numbers of people living to 100 within specific populations, Dan Buettner says that "by adopting the right lifestyle we could add at least ten good years and suffer a fraction of the diseases that kill us prematurely. This could mean an extra *quality* decade of life!"[11] It is part of our experience of being human to want to live long, happy and healthy lives, but when we look at lifestyle and illness in the developed world today, we seem to be living in ways that contrast starkly with our desires for longevity and a disease-free life.

› Obesity and sedentary lifestyles

We have become increasingly inactive in our daily lives as technology has brought many improvements and labor-saving devices that mean we don't have to work as hard for necessities such as food and shelter.

Desk jobs, computer time and television have contributed to a new pattern of living—the sedentary lifestyle. In this situation where input regularly exceeds output, weight gain is an unavoidable outcome. Obesity is now the single most preventable cause of disease in men and women.[12] Excess weight contributes to the development of many of the major diseases we experience today. Obesity is now as damaging to health as smoking.

Chronic disease and illness are not a natural part of the aging process despite the statistics that tell us disease rates are on the rise.

A low-fat, high-fiber, plant-based diet is effective in reducing insulin resistance, enhancing weight control and reversing the diabetic condition.

› Cardiovascular disease

As a total health approach, lifestyle medicine has gathered momentum over the past decades as research has increased our understanding of the role nutrition and exercise play in health. No research effort has contributed more to understanding the links between lifestyle and cardiovascular disease, for example, than the Framingham Heart Study, which has followed three generations of people.

A report from the Framingham Heart Study puts it like this: "Over the years, careful monitoring of the Framingham Study population has led to the identification of the major cardiovascular disease risk factors—high blood pressure, high blood cholesterol, smoking, obesity, diabetes, and physical inactivity—as well as a great deal of valuable information on the effects of related factors such as blood triglyceride and HDL cholesterol levels, age, gender, and psychosocial issues."[13]

› Diabetes

It is clear that lifestyle factors such as obesity are pre-causal to many of the chronic and degenerative diseases that we consider part of the aging process, but it is also a key factor in the development of illnesses at any time in the lifespan, with a particularly good example being the onset of type 2 diabetes. Dr Neal Barnard, through his research into the reversal of this disease, has shown that a low-fat, high-fiber, plant-based diet is effective in reducing insulin resistance, enhancing weight control and reversing the diabetic condition. It is also protective for those who are at risk for diabetes and results are further enhanced by the addition of a suitable exercise program.[14]

A new way of thinking about medicine and health care

Lifestyle medicine changes our understanding of what it means to be in optimal health today and how we respond to our society's epidemic of chronic disease. It provides a total-health approach that looks at every area of a person's life in response to disease and puts the patient at the center. Many of the principles of lifestyle medicine are simple, logical and familiar to the ear, considering the human body as a unique system with a natural capacity to heal given the right lifestyle choices. To a significant degree, our lifestyle choices determine our state of health.

This new way of understanding medicine and health care is now our best way forward to optimal health. As the research indicates, prevention and reversal of our modern chronic diseases is preferable to disease management. Shifting our thinking from simply controlling illness, lifestyle medicine offers choices that are the key to optimal health. As inventor and visionary Thomas Edison put it, "The doctor of the future will give no medicine, but will interest patients in the care of the human frame, in diet, and in the cause and prevention of disease."

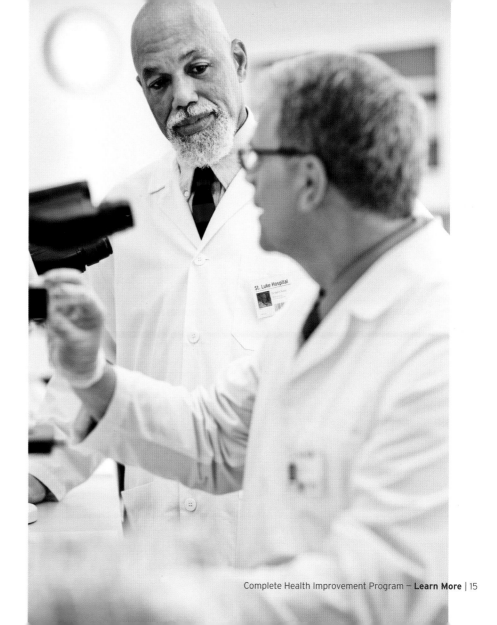

Chapter One References

1. Australian Institute of Health and Welfare (2010), "Australia's health 2010; the tenth biennial report of the Australian Institute of Health and Welfare," Cat no Aus 73.

2. Ossler, W (1928), "The prevalence of coronary heart disease in North America."

3. Miniño A M, et al (2011), "Deaths: Final data for 2008," National Vital Statistics Reports, Vol 59 No 10, National Center for Health Statistics; see also Centers for Disease Control (2012), *National Vital Statistics Reports*, Vol 60 No 4.

4. World Health Organization (2011), "Cardiovascular Disease Fact Sheet No 317," <www.who.int/mediacentre/factsheets/fs317/en/index.html>.

5. ibid.

6. World Health Organization (2011), "Diabetes Fact Sheet No 312," <www.who.int/mediacentre/factsheets/fs312/en/index.html>.

7. World Health Organization (2011), "Hypertension Fact Sheet," <www.searo.who.int/linkfiles/non_communicable_diseases_hypertension-fs.pdf>.

8. Centers for Disease Control and Prevention (2011), "Diabetes: Successes and opportunities for population-based prevention and control."

9. Holman, H (2004), "Chronic Disease—The Need for a New Clinical Education," *Journal of the American Medical Association*, Vol 292 No 9, pages 1057-1059; GDP: Employee Benefit Research Institute estimate from Centers for Medicare and Medicaid Services and US Department of Commerce (2005-2015 projected).

10. For the researched background and confirmation of Dr Burkitt's statement, see:
    › Yusuf, S, et al (2004), "Effect of potentially modifiable risk factors associated with myocardial infarction in 52 countries (the INTERHEART study): case-control study," *Lancet*, Vol 364 No 9438, pages 937-52.
    › Ornish, D, et al (1990), "Can lifestyle changes reverse coronary heart disease? The Lifestyle Heart Trial," *Lancet*, Vol 336 No 8708, pages 129-33.
    › Esselstyn, C B, Jr (1999), "Updating a 12-year experience with arrest and reversal therapy for coronary heart disease (an overdue requiem for palliative cardiology)," *American Journal of Cardiology*, Vol 84 No 3, pages 339-41, A8.

11. Buettner, D (2008), *The Blue Zone: lessons for living longer from the people who have lived the longest*, National Geographic Society, page 2.

12. Egger G, Binns A, Rossner S (2011), *Lifestyle Medicine: Managing diseases of lifestyle in the 21st century*, McGraw-Hill Australia, page 12.

13. Framingham Heart Study (2012), <www.framinghamheartstudy.org>.

14. Barnard, N D, et al (2006), "A low-fat vegan diet improves glycemic control and cardiovascular risk factors in a randomized clinical trial in individuals with type 2 diabetes," *Diabetes Care*, Vol 29 No 8, pages 1777-83.

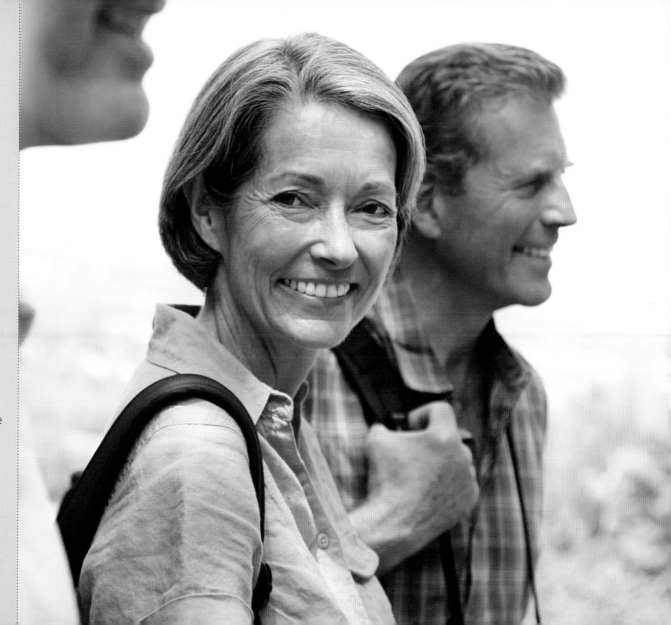

KEY POINTS

› Modern medicine has developed many remarkable treatments and cures.

› However, modern lifestyles have also significantly contributed to a growing burden of chronic disease.

› Understanding that today's chronic diseases are largely lifestyle related, we realize they must be preventable and potentially reversible by better lifestyle choices.

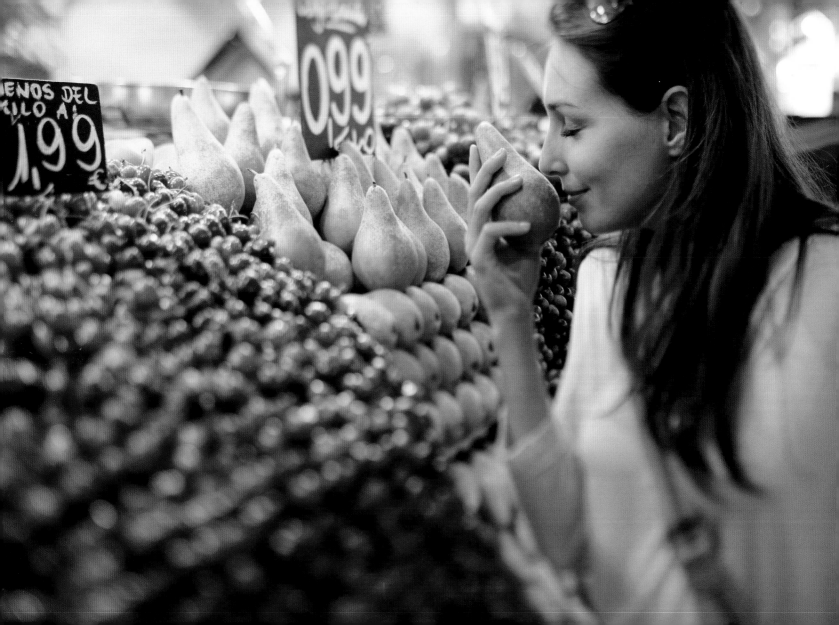

Chapter Two

Lifestyle is the Best Medicine

Imagine enjoying not just good health but optimal health and wellbeing! Lifestyle medicine puts the power of health back into our own hands. With its solid research base and "whole-health" approach, it is the best medicine for preventing and reversing disease as it responds fully to the causes of disease and the demands of modern living, and helps us re-discover who we are as healthy, happy people.

Optimal health as a way of life

The lifestyle medicine approach works best because it encourages us to expand our under-standing of good health from being merely an absence of symptoms, to knowing we can achieve and maintain optimal health by living best-practice health principles. Optimal health is the essence of a good life. The World Health Organization (WHO) defines optimal health as "inclusive of physical, social, psychological, emotional and spiritual wellbeing." Optimal health is a way of living that helps us realize our potential, supporting quantity of life (longevity) and quality of life.

The science of lifestyle and disease prevention

Over the past few decades, many scientific stud-ies have reinforced the role of lifestyle in health and disease. Lifestyle medicine has scientifically proven research as its foundation, and a range of important worldwide studies have provided insights into the nature of disease, risk factors and the ways in which lifestyle can be modified for positive health outcomes. It has been an exciting time in health research, as discoveries have been made that can dramatically influence the course of disease, with restoration of optimal health as its goal.

Optimal health is a way of living that helps us realize our potential, supporting quantity of life (longevity) and quality of life.

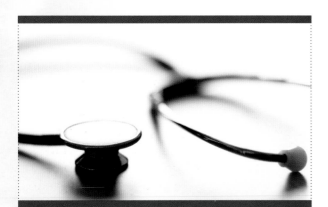

Lifestyle Medicine:
A TEXTBOOK DEFINITION

Lifestyle medicine is a total-health approach that has its foundation in "the application of environmental, behavioral, medical and motivational principles to the management of lifestyle-related health problems in a clinical setting" and offers us a map with which we can navigate the "proper treatment of chronic disease."[1] When we add the concepts of self-care and self-management, a picture emerges of an empowered patient with a different set of beliefs about health and what it is to be well.

Some of the most significant lifestyle and disease prevention research studies are:

› Established in 1949, the Framingham Heart Study is a joint study between Boston University and the National Heart, Lung, and Blood Institute, USA. This three-generational study has provided tangible evidence of the role lifestyle and diet play particularly in coronary heart disease. This groundbreaking study was the first of its kind and continues to be one of the most highly regarded studies into lifestyle and disease today. [2]

› In the 1960s, Dr Lester Breslow, the Public Health Director of Alameda County in northern California, studied the lifestyle habits, illnesses and deaths of 7000 adults over a period of nine years. He found seven health habits that correlated most successfully with life expectancy:

- Regular meals, without snacking

- Daily breakfast

- Regular exercise

- Adequate sleep

- No smoking

- Moderate weight

- No or limited alcohol

Dr Breslow found that those who practised fewer than four health habits when compared to those who practised all seven health habits had four times as many deaths. Moreover he found that 45-year-old males practising six to seven health habits could expect to live 11.5 years longer than those practising three or less. And this research found that "those who practised all seven health habits had the health status of those 30 years younger who observed none."[3]

› The famous EPIC Norfolk Study—based at Cambridge University in the UK—enrolled 20,000 adults without known cardiovascular disease or cancer. During the next 11 years, they recorded almost 2000 deaths from this group, then correlated them with four simple health habits:

- Smoking
- Alcohol consumption
- Fruit and vegetable consumption
- Physical activity

The study found a four-fold difference in mortality risk between those who made healthy choices in relation to all four and those who chose poorly. The difference was equivalent to 14 years of life. The authors concluded: "This study suggests that even small differences in lifestyle can have a profound effect on longevity and health."[4]

› The role of diet in disease was the subject of a study carried out by Cornell University, Oxford University and the University of Beijing, with Dr T Colin Campbell as principal investigator. This was a long-term observational study, including 6500 adults from different parts of China. This research found more than 8000 statistically significant associations between various dietary factors and disease. Importantly, it also showed that through a healthy diet of plant-based whole foods, many diseases are much less prevalent—a significant finding that illustrated the vital role of diet in health.

While the researchers noted generally low levels of heart disease and cancer among study participants, they found a significant correlation with the range of cholesterol levels across the population studied. Those at the upper end of their relatively low cholesterol range had markedly more heart disease, more cancer and more diabetes than those at the lower end. While eating animal products largely influences blood cholesterol levels, the researchers were surprised that "even small intakes of animal products were powerfully related to increases in heart disease, cancer and diabetes."[5]

Another population group that has been the subject of extensive health studies is members of the Seventh-day Adventist Church. Recognized by Dan Buettner in his *Blue Zones* project among the world's "longevity all-stars"—particularly the church members in Loma Linda, California—research in a number of countries has found church members consistently living between six and 10 years longer than the general population in which they live.[6] With common lifestyle recommendations and practices but a variety of dietary choices, this identifiable population has been recognized as having great potential as research subjects, giving rise to more than 300 scientific publications.

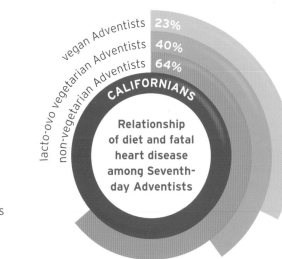

vegan Adventists 23%
lacto-ovo vegetarian Adventists 40%
non-vegetarian Adventists 64%
CALIFORNIANS

Relationship of diet and fatal heart disease among Seventh-day Adventists

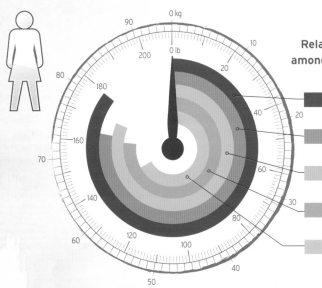

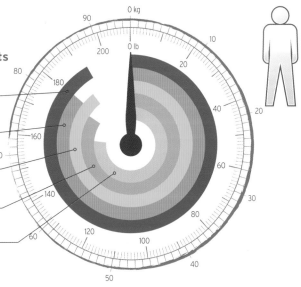

Relationship of diet and average weight among Californian Seventh-day Adventists

From the Adventist Health Study 2

NON-VEGETARIAN
F 180Lb (82kg)   M 193Lb (87kg)

SEMI-VEGETARIAN
F 164Lb (74kg)   M 181Lb (82kg)

PESCO-VEGETARIAN
F 171Lb (77kg)   M 188Lb (85kg)

LACTO-OVO VEGETARIAN
F 161Lb (73kg)   M 177Lb (80kg)

TOTAL VEGETARIAN
F 141Lb (64kg)   M 161Lb (73kg)

For example, in the California-based Adventist Health Study 1, researchers found that Adventist meat-eaters had 300 per cent more fatal heart disease than those following a solely plant-based diet. Expanding the Californian study to include some 97,000 Seventh-day Adventist church members from the United States and Canada, researchers for the Adventist Health Study 2 found that Adventists following a plant-based diet had the best health outcomes in the areas of weight, cholesterol, hypertension and diabetes when compared with church members who differentiated themselves primarily by consumption of animal products.[7]

NON-VEGETARIAN
Includes meat regularly in their diet

SEMI-VEGETARIAN
Has at least one meal a week with meat

PESCO-VEGETARIAN
Includes seafood in their diet but no meat

LACTO-OVO VEGETARIAN
Includes dairy products and eggs in their diet

TOTAL VEGETARIAN
Excludes all animal products—including eggs, dairy, and honey—from their diet.

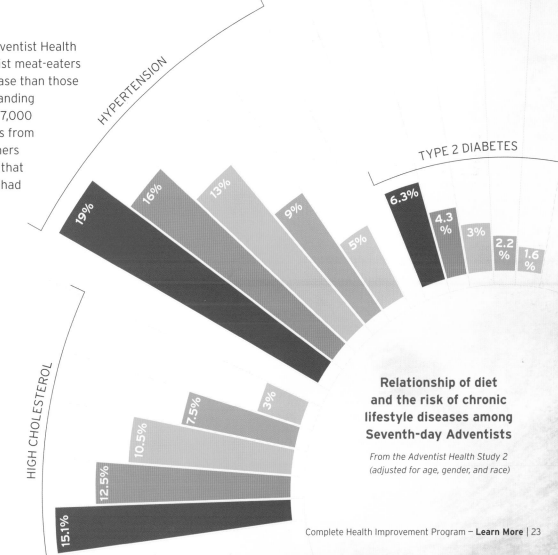

HYPERTENSION

TYPE 2 DIABETES

HIGH CHOLESTEROL

Relationship of diet and the risk of chronic lifestyle diseases among Seventh-day Adventists

From the Adventist Health Study 2 (adjusted for age, gender, and race)

Hypertension: 19% | 16% | 13% | 9% | 5%

Type 2 Diabetes: 6.3% | 4.3% | 3% | 2.2% | 1.6%

High Cholesterol: 15.1% | 12.5% | 10.5% | 7.5% | 3%

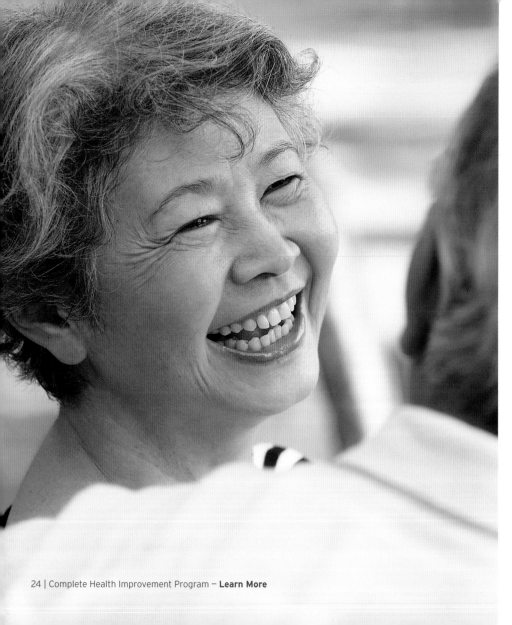

The science of disease reversal

While each of these studies—and many more—have demonstrated the role of lifestyle choices in the development or prevention of chronic diseases, other medical practitioners explored the effect of these same general principles to repair and reverse the health damage lifestyle choices may have caused to their patients' lives.

› One of the pioneers of lifestyle medicine for disease reversal is Dr Dean Ornish. Over 35 years, Dr Ornish has developed several integrative programs that have been proven effective in reversing heart disease; slowing, stopping or reversing the progression of prostate cancer; and influencing aging. Beyond cancer, heart disease and diabetes, Dr Ornish's studies have also considered lifestyle conditions such as high blood pressure, cholesterol, obesity and gene expression and, without exception, lifestyle factors have been shown to play a critical part in disease development and response.[8]

In his most famous study, Dr Ornish took 48 cardiac patients and instructed half of them to follow a very low-fat vegetarian diet. The control group received the standard care instructions on how to lose weight, exercise and follow a "balanced" diet, with modest meat restriction. After one year, the vegetarian group had lowered their total cholesterol by 24 per cent and 82 per cent of their atherosclerotic plaques had begun to "melt down." In the standard care group, however, the total cholesterol had dropped only 5 per cent and 53 per cent of the lesions had worsened.[9] A Newsweek article reported these results in 1998: "[Ornish] has proved, scientifically, that people can open their blocked arteries without drugs or surgery. Instead of splitting people's torsos to replumb their hearts, he guides them through a rigorous lifestyle program."[10]

> Dr Caldwell Esselstyn Jr has been another long-term advocate for the power of lifestyle modification in patient treatment. His published research showed that coronary disease could be reversed through diet and lifestyle changes and his work has influenced many other studies in this area. His program—

with its focus on a plant-based, oil-free diet—has been seen to not only reverse heart disease, but also helped patients remain symptom-free for life.[11]

Dr Esselstyn took extreme heart disease patients and instructed them in a very low-fat vegetarian diet of simple plant-based foods as grown, with no animal products. His patients experienced remarkable results. In his book, he describes his 20-year follow up with his patients, many of whom had been given only six months to live by their cardiologists.[12] Drawing on his experiences and proven treatments, Dr Esselstyn states: "For the minority of heart patients, specifically those in the midst of heart attacks or acute coronary syndromes, stents or coronary artery bypass may be lifesaving. For the rest, none of the present therapies targets the cause: the Western diet."[13]

> Another proven lifestyle intervention program that has resulted in demonstrable health

"Instead of splitting people's torsos to replumb their hearts, he guides them through a rigorous lifestyle program."

benefits in the lives of its many participants is that of which this book is part—the Complete Health Improvement Program (CHIP), previously known as the Coronary Health Improvement Project. Since its launch around the world in 1987, tens of thousands of participants have been able to experience improvements in their health status through CHIP. Adding to the many personal success stories, the results of blood tests and health assessments conducted with participants before and after this program have given scientifically measurable indications that significant health problems can be reversed as a result of lifestyle change.

Analyzing the results from more than 5000 participants who participated in CHIP between 2006 and 2009, researchers have found that "significant reductions in body weight and CVD [cardiovascular disease] risk factors can be achieved through a lifestyle intervention program delivered in a community setting by volunteers. Furthermore, those with the greatest risk benefited the most."[14]

Since its launch around the world in 1987, tens of thousands of participants have been able to experience improvements in their health status through CHIP.

The combined approach of lifestyle medicine

This growing weight of research and medical evidence demonstrates the effectiveness of lifestyle medicine for both disease prevention and reversal. The causes of chronic disease are a combination of many lifestyle factors, so it stands to reason that the response to any disease requires a multi-factorial approach: "Narrow attention on single risk factors and their association with disease led to clinical recommendations focused primarily on managing these individual risk factors, particularly raised blood pressure and cholesterol."[15] Lifestyle medicine shifts the emphasis from a single risk factor to the combined risk by addressing all aspects of a patient's lifestyle that contribute to illness. There is no single answer or magical treatment that will restore health or improve a patient's disease. The body is a complex organism with highly individualized responses and patterns, and it needs to be seen as a "whole-person" system with a unique set of needs for care.

Differences observed between traditional/conventional and lifestyle medicine approaches in primary care[16]

TRADITIONAL/CONVENTIONAL MEDICINE	LIFESTYLE MEDICINE
› Treats individual risk factors	› Treats lifestyle causes
› Patient is a passive recipient of care	› Patient is an active partner in care
› Patient is not required to make big changes	› Patient is required to make big changes
› Treatment is often short term	› Treatment is always long term
› Responsibility is on the clinician	› Responsibility is also on the patient
› Medication is often the 'end' treatment	› Medication may be needed but emphasis is on lifestyle change
› Emphasizes diagnosis and prescription	› Emphasizes motivation and compliance
› Goal is disease management	› Goal is primary/secondary/tertiary prevention
› Less consideration of environment	› More consideration of environment
› Side effects are balanced by benefits	› Side effects that impact on lifestyle require greater attention
› Involves other medical specialties	› Involves allied health professionals
› Doctors generally operate independently, on a one-to-one basis	› Doctors frequently work with patients in groups with other health professionals

The empowered patient

Patient-centered care is of central concern to lifestyle medicine. In contrast to an "expert" writing a script for a pill and similar treatments—all of which happen *to* a patient—the patient is an active partner in the lifestyle medicine model. The emphasis is on responsibility and typically requires a long-term personal commitment for lasting benefits. Although medication might be used, it may be considered more as an aid to lifestyle changes, to quickly manage risk factors while addressing underlying lifestyle behaviors, not as the primary way to obtain results. In patient-centered care, the causes of illness are discussed and jointly understood between the practitioner and the patient. Information, inspiration and motivation are the keys to any consultation and any lifestyle change.

There is an understanding that healing occurs from inside to outside and the importance of self-healing and commitment to change is both a co-created and co-managed approach. Lifestyle medicine brings a sense of power and control back to the individual that encourages the willingness to change. Empowerment supports better health outcomes for individuals, fosters better health and wellbeing in communities, and encourages responsible thinking at large. It is a vital part of a bigger discussion about community health, the environment and sustainability, and affects public and personal health in daily life.

Relearning health

With its focus on consultation and life planning, lifestyle medicine is an effective education tool that can directly influence the health status of patients. Health literacy—"the degree to which individuals have the capacity to obtain, process and understand basic health information and services needed to make appropriate health decisions"[17]—is considered one of the most important and least understood factors in health management. The focus of lifestyle medicine on health education and policy is an important area that cannot be overlooked.

Learning to make changes to lifestyle can begin with making more conscious choices in everyday life. When next shopping for food ask: "Is this food an investment in my health, or at the expense of my health?" Simple actions in

"Is this food an investment in my health, or at the expense of my health?"

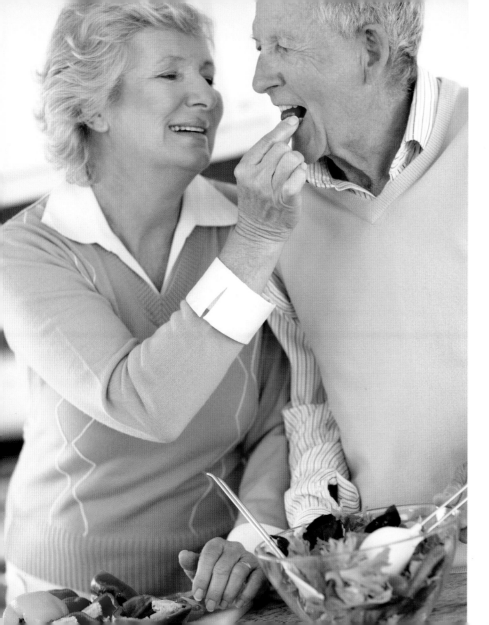

everyday life can—and do—make a difference to lifestyle and will help us make the changes we need to make in order to live happy, healthy lives. We want to live long and we want to live well. If we look to the lessons about longevity offered in *The Blue Zone* study we find: "The world's longevity all-stars not only live longer, they also tend to live better. They have strong connections with their family and friends. They're active. They wake up in the morning knowing that they have a purpose, and the world in turn, reacts to them in a way that propels them along. An overwhelming majority of them still enjoy life. And there's not a grump in the bunch."[18] Each and every day, lifestyle medicine offers both a way to optimal health and a possibility for healing the damage our lifestyle has created.

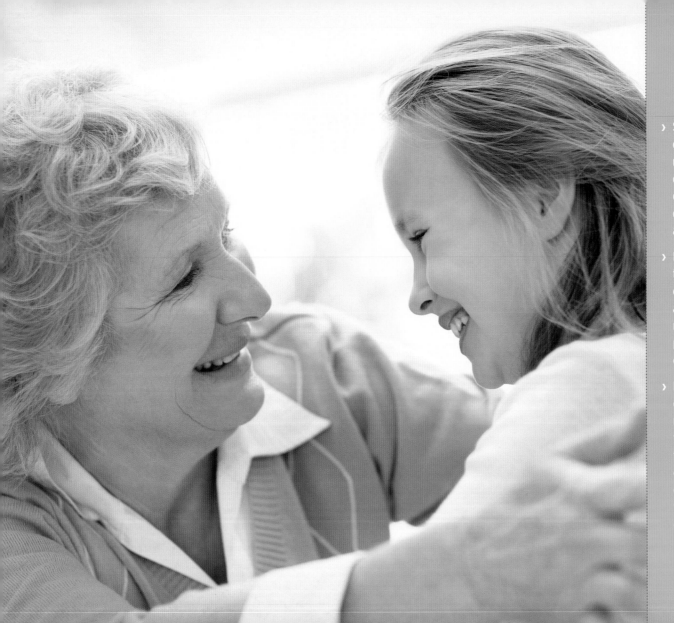

Chapter Two References

1   Egger G, Binns A, Rossner S (2011), *Lifestyle Medicine–Managing diseases of lifestyle in the 21st century*, McGraw-Hill Australia Pty Ltd, page 1.

2   Framingham Heart Study (1948-), <http://www.framinghamheartstudy.org/>, accessed March 2012.

3   Belloc, N B and L Breslow (1972), "Relationship of physical health status and health practices," *Preventative Medicine*, Vol 1 No 3, pages 409–21; see also Breslow, L and J E Enstrom (1980), "Persistence of health habits and their relationship to mortality," *Preventative Medicine*, Vol 9 No 4, page 469–83.

4   Khaw, K T, et al (2008), "Combined impact of health behaviours and mortality in men and women: the EPIC-Norfolk prospective population study," *PLoS Medicine*, Vol 5 No 1, page e12.

5   Campbell, T C, B Parpia, and J Chen (1998), "Diet, lifestyle, and the etiology of coronary artery disease: the Cornell China study," *American Journal of Cardiology*, Vol 82 No 10B, pages 18T–21T.

6   Berkel, J and F de Waard (1983), "Mortality pattern and life expectancy of Seventh-day Adventists in the Netherlands," *International Journal of Epidemiology*, Vol 12 No 4, pages 455–9; Jedrychowski, W, et al (1985), "Survival rates among Seventh-day Adventists compared with the general population in Poland," *Scandinavian Journal of Social Medicine*, Vol 13 No 2, page 49–52; Fraser, G E and D J Shavlik (2001), "Ten years of life: Is it a matter of choice?" *Archive of Internal Medicine*, Vol 161 No 13, pages 1645–52.

7   Fraser, G E (2009), "Vegetarian diets: what do we know of their effects on common chronic diseases?" *American Journal of Clinical Nutrition*, Vol 89 No 5, pages 1607S–1612S; Tonstad, S, et al (2009), "Type of vegetarian diet, body weight, and prevalence of type 2 diabetes," *Diabetes Care*, Vol 32 No 5, pages 791–6.

8   Ornish, D (1995), *Dr Dean Ornish's Program for Reversing Heart Disease: The Only System Scientifically Proven to Reverse Heart Disease Without Drugs or Surgery*, Ivy Books.

9   Ornish, D, et al (1998), "Intensive lifestyle changes for reversal of coronary heart disease," *Journal of the American Medical Association*, Vol 280 No 23, pages 2001–7.

10 Cowley G, "How Dean Ornish is Shaking Up Medicine," *Newsweek*, March 16, 1998.

11 Esselstyn, C B Jr, et al (1995), "A strategy to arrest and reverse coronary artery disease: a 5-year longitudinal study of a single physician's practice," *Journal of Family Practice*, Vol 41 No 6, pages 560–8.

12 Esselstyn, C B Jr (2007), *Prevent and Reverse Heart Disease: The Revolutionary, Scientifically Proven, Nutrition-based Cure*, Penguin Group.

13 Esselstyn, C B Jr (2010), "Is the present therapy for coronary artery disease the radical mastectomy of the twenty-first century?" *American Journal of Cardiology*, Vol 106, pages 902–4.

14 Rankin, P, D Morton, H Diehl, et al (2012), "Effectiveness of a Volunteer-Delivered Lifestyle Modification Program for Reducing Cardiovascular Disease Risk Factors," *American Journal of Cardiology*, Vol 109 No 1, pages 82–6.

15 Egger, op cit, page 16.

16 Adapted from Egger, page 5.

17 Ratzan and Parker, 2000, quoted by Egger, ibid, page 53.

18 Buettner, D (2008), *The Blue Zone: Lessons for living longer from the people who have lived the longest*, National Geographic Society, Washington, page 227.

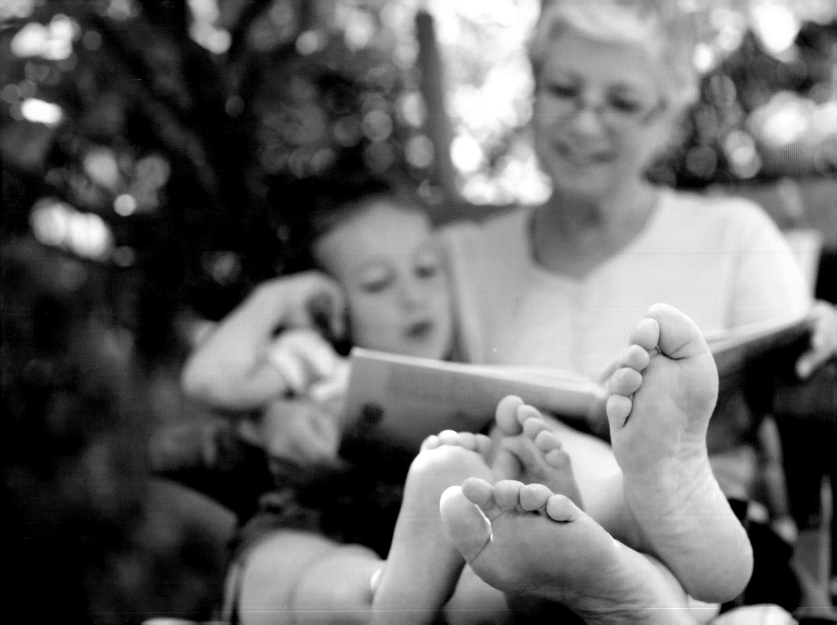

Chapter Three

The Optimal Lifestyle

New York journalist A J Jacobs has become a successful author by chronicling his life experiments, taking an idea or set of ideas and seeing how they play out in his own life. In his 2012 book, *Drop Dead Healthy: One Man's Humble Quest for Bodily Perfection*, Jacobs sets out to try many different health ideas, recommendations and prescriptions over a two-year period. While also exploring some of the more bizarre and extreme of health ideas, his experiments are based on medical research, as far as possible, and his book highlights the difficulty of sorting out all the different and competing health advice we receive all the time. However, he comes to the simple summary: "Most health advice can be summed up in five words: *Eat less, move more, relax.*"[1]

It sounds simplistic but it is not so far from the truth. Belying the mountain of medical research reported regularly in the media and the plethora of health products and programs marketed to us, the core principles of healthy lifestyle are simple and effective in reducing risks and potentially reversing the full range of chronic disease. Unlike the "diets," "plans" and programs aimed at specific illnesses—for example, "cancer-reducing," "diabetes-controlling," "liver-cleansing" or "heart-strengthening"—the optimal lifestyle offers the best response to any and all of these diseases, and the best prescription for healthy living.

While we might be rightly skeptical of a "one-size-fits-all" response to chronic lifestyle diseases, the effectiveness of lifestyle medicine makes sense when we understand the body processes that underlie all chronic diseases.

The optimal lifestyle offers the best response to any and all of these diseases, and the best prescription for healthy living.

Introducing inflammation

If you have ever had a splinter in your finger, you might have noticed that the area around the splinter turned red, began to swell and became increasingly painful. Your body's response to the injury and presence of the splinter was inflammation, which is the body's immune system working effectively to combat bacteria or viruses that might have been introduced to the body by this intrusion. When the splinter was removed, the inflammation should have soon subsided and your body quietly went about healing itself.

A similar process happens throughout our body when it is threatened in different ways by attackers to the body's healthy and natural functions. Poor lifestyle choices can lead to an ongoing, low-level inflammation throughout the body, which in turn creates a chronic state of mild distress within your body, increasing the risk of chronic diseases.

Poor lifestyle choices can lead to an ongoing, low-level inflammation throughout the body.

Lifestyle factors such as smoking, a lack of activity, stress, obesity and what we eat can all drive this chronic low-level inflammation. This, in turn, affects the lining of our blood vessels throughout the body and also our normal metabolic functioning. Instead of a relatively

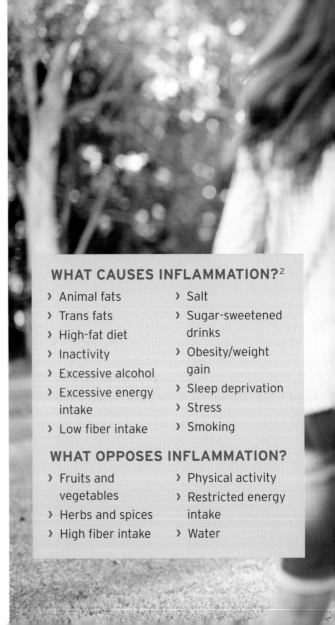

WHAT CAUSES INFLAMMATION?[2]

> Animal fats
> Trans fats
> High-fat diet
> Inactivity
> Excessive alcohol
> Excessive energy intake
> Low fiber intake
> Salt
> Sugar-sweetened drinks
> Obesity/weight gain
> Sleep deprivation
> Stress
> Smoking

WHAT OPPOSES INFLAMMATION?

> Fruits and vegetables
> Herbs and spices
> High fiber intake
> Physical activity
> Restricted energy intake
> Water

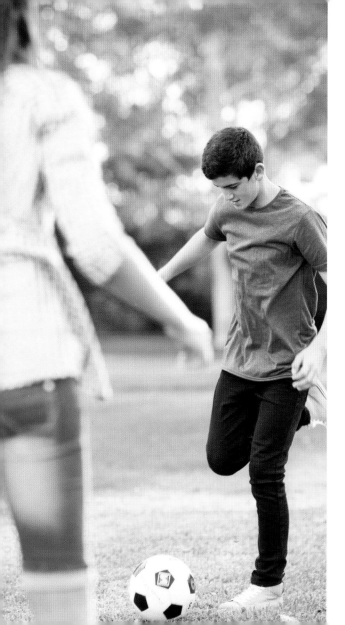

short-term inflammation and consequent healing, we end up with a confused metabolism and inflamed blood vessels, eventually leading to insulin resistance—a precursor to diabetes[3]—heart and arterial diseases,[4] increased cancer risks, Alzheimer's disease[5] and other chronic diseases.

What is "oxidative stress"?

Another closely related process that is being increasingly linked to chronic diseases is called "oxidative stress", which is a principal cause of inflammation, infection, cancer, cardiovascular disorders and even aging itself.[6] Natural body processes and unhealthy lifestyle choices create "free radicals" within our body. These are harmful substances that damage otherwise healthy molecules within our cells. Because they are unstable molecules, they seek to bond with other molecules, damaging these healthy molecules in the process. Too much of this kind of damage causes stress within the cells and causes the body's immune system to respond, leading to inflammation.

The body's protectors against free radicals are known as antioxidants. Antioxidants are molecules that connect with free radicals, preventing them from doing damage to other molecules within the body.

In simple terms, oxidative stress is an imbalance between free radicals and antioxidants in the body. This can be contributed to by an excess of substances, metabolism of which results in the production of free radicals—such as unhealthy foods, alcohol or cigarette smoke—or a deficiency in substances with antioxidant properties or activities, such as fruits, vegetables and physical activity. The key to generating oxidative stress is an excess of substances and behaviors that promote free radical production.

A compounding problem

One of the primary sites of this chronic low-level inflammation is the body's more than 60,000 miles (about 100,000 kilometers) of blood vessels. The health of the body's circulatory system is key to many aspects of our overall health. When circulation is impaired, insufficient oxygen is delivered around the body—known as hypoxia—in turn impairing the various bodily functions and processes, and increasing risks of disease and loss of function.

The main contributor to poor circulation is atherosclerosis, commonly known as "narrowing and hardening of the arteries." It has been described as a "silent killer" because it grows slowly and imperceptibly—and all too often the first "symptom" is sudden death, usually by heart attack.

We're born with clean and flexible arteries and they should really stay that way over time. But the common pattern today is that cholesterol, fats and calcium have already formed plaques that narrow our arterial lumen by some 20 per cent by the time we are 20 years of age.[7] That this kind of disease is so far progressed in young people might take us by surprise but autopsies

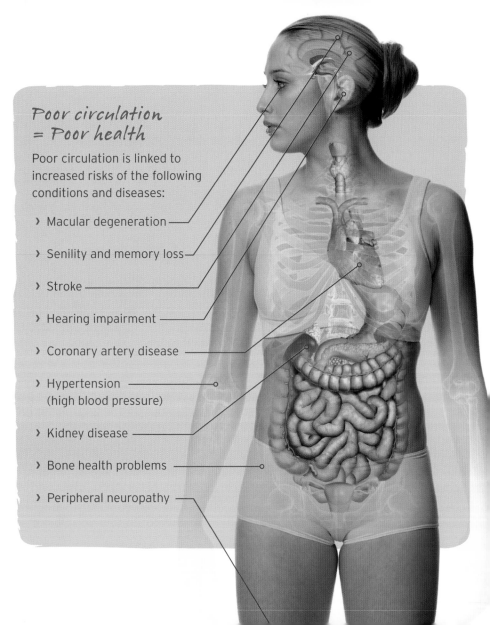

Poor circulation = Poor health

Poor circulation is linked to increased risks of the following conditions and diseases:

› Macular degeneration

› Senility and memory loss

› Stroke

› Hearing impairment

› Coronary artery disease

› Hypertension (high blood pressure)

› Kidney disease

› Bone health problems

› Peripheral neuropathy

conducted on United States soldiers who died in the Korean War in the early 1950s demonstrated this sobering reality. The average age of the soldiers examined was just 22, but 77 per cent had significantly narrowed arteries. Interestingly, similar tests on Korean soldiers—who had grown up with quite different lifestyles and diets—rarely found the disease even in those twice this age.[8] With the increasing adoption of the "Western" diet around the world, similar comparisons would be less likely to be as noticeable today.

While atherosclerosis and significant arterial blockages can occur or potentially be avoided at any time throughout our lives, typically, by the time many of us are 45 years of age, plaque can have grown to the point that it narrows our arterial lumen by about 50 per cent. And by 70 years of age, many live with 90 per cent narrowing of their arteries, leaving only 10 per cent opening for blood to flow through.

Apart from the chronic inflammation discussed above, the risk factors for atherosclerosis are primarily diet-related, particularly cholesterol. Cholesterol levels in our blood are dictated largely by our food choices, which can work to both raise and lower our cholesterol. Of particular interest is the level of LDL ("bad") cholesterol, which in its oxidized form is key to the formation of atherosclerotic plaques.

Cholesterol levels in our blood are dictated largely by our food choices, which can work to both raise and lower our cholesterol.

NITRIC OXIDE

Nitric oxide is a molecule produced by a number of different cells in the body, but its production in vascular blood vessels is particularly important in the regulation of blood flow. The inner lining of blood vessels, known as the endothelium, produces nitric oxide, which signals the vessels to relax and expand, ensuring easy blood flow. Nitric oxide also has an anti-thrombotic effect, which helps stop blood platelets from sticking to the blood vessel walls, and also an anti-inflammatory effect, helping prevent damage to the blood vessel linings. Conditions such as atherosclerosis and diabetes, which can cause damage to the blood vessel linings, can contribute to a decreased production of nitric oxide, causing vascular complications and increasing the risk of heart disease.[9]

What is Atherosclerosis?

The main contributor to poor circulation is atherosclerosis, commonly known as "narrowing and hardening of the arteries."

Typically, by the time many of us are 45 years of age, plaque can have grown to the point that it narrows our arterial lumen by about 50 per cent. And by 70 years of age, many live with 90 per cent narrowing of their arteries, leaving only 10 per cent opening for blood to flow through.

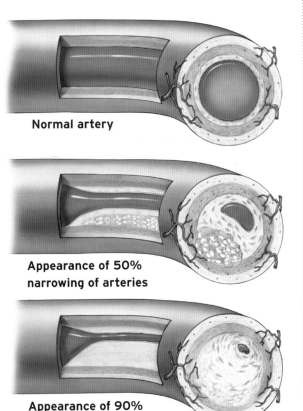

Normal artery

Appearance of 50% narrowing of arteries

Appearance of 90% narrowing of arteries

The rich "Western" diet and our lifestyle in general can injure the endothelium—the innermost lining of our arteries. As this becomes more permeable to oxidized LDL cholesterol, inflammatory processes are set up that may hinder adequate nitric oxide production, which is needed to protect these inner most linings to keep them elastic.

As early as 1978, Dr Jeremiah Stamler, a well-known cardiologist, concluded from the evidence available at that time that it was "reasonable and sound to designate 'rich' diet as a primary, essential, necessary cause of the current epidemic of premature atherosclerotic disease raging in the Western industrialized countries."[10]

Attacking the heart

While we often talk about heart attacks and heart disease, there is usually nothing wrong with the heart muscle, the myocardium. Instead, the problem usually resides inside the coronary arteries—arteries supplying blood to the heart muscle—that deliver oxygen- and nutrient-rich blood to the heart muscle to keep it nourished and in good running order.

As the coronary arteries progressively narrow and harden, the evolving disease is free of symptoms for a long time. The first common symptom, such as chest pain (angina pectoris), often appears only after some 70 per cent narrowing of the coronary arteries has made it difficult to deliver the oxygen needed by the heart muscle, especially during exercise or other exertion.

In this way, angina is an early warning sign of the larger and serious health problem. When a coronary artery becomes fully blocked, this prevents the flow of blood to part of the heart muscle, which begins to starve of oxygen and then to die. The narrower the artery, the greater the risk of it being blocked by a rupture in the plaque-lined artery wall or a blood clot, which is also a greater risk when circulation is impaired.

About 10 per cent of heart attacks result from blockages directly related to the accumulated hard plaques. The greater risks—and those leading to as many as 90 per cent of heart attacks—are those of softer plaques, deposits of which are linked to higher cholesterol and are more unstable, so more likely to rupture and block blood flow to the heart muscle.[11] These dangerous soft plaques often go unnoticed, even in angiograms.

The conventional medical treatments for these medical emergencies are the extremely invasive open-heart bypass surgery—using replacement vessels to "bypass" the blocked or nearly blocked coronary arteries—or arterial stents to reopen blocked arteries, and ongoing medication to manage and reduce risk factors.

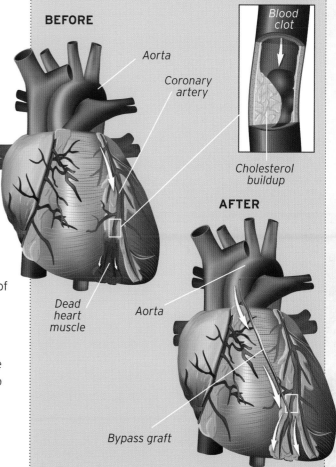

Coronary Artery Bypass

BEFORE

Aorta

Coronary artery

Blood clot

Cholesterol buildup

AFTER

Dead heart muscle

Aorta

Bypass graft

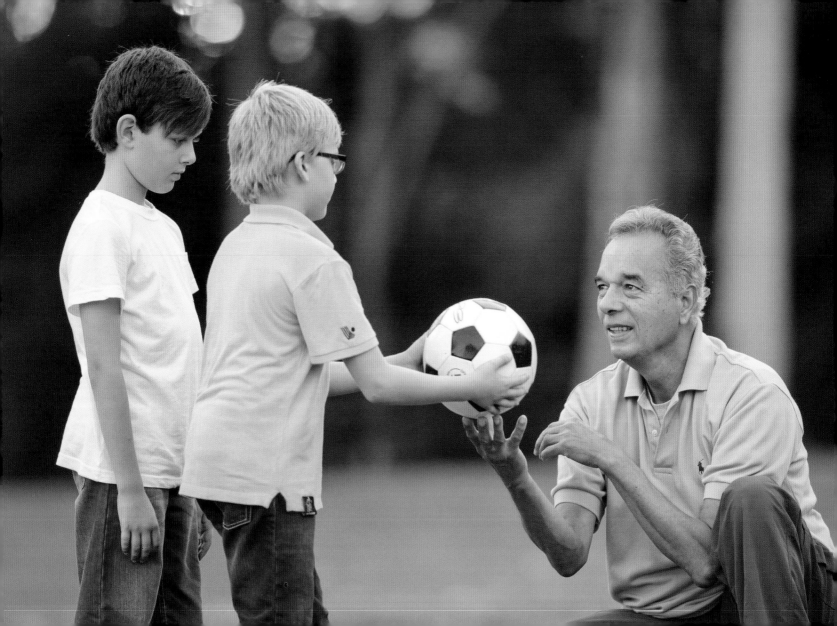

Beyond the heart

Of course, the build up of atherosclerotic plaque is not limited to coronary arteries. The same process can affect our arteries in all parts of the body. This impaired circulation can cause or contribute to degenerative and chronic disease throughout the body:

› When it affects the cerebral and carotid arteries, where the narrowing and hardening is associated with strokes, hearing loss, visual loss, macular degeneration of the eyes, senility, and also in part with Alzheimer's.

› When it affects the arteries providing blood to the kidneys, we have to be concerned about high blood pressure and kidney disease.

› When it affects the blood flow to the joints, we see increased risks of avascular necrosis, which is associated with hip fractures.

› When it affects the penile arteries, we have to be concerned with erectile dysfunction and impotence. Impotence may also be a first sign of a larger problem and has been described as "the canary in the coal mine"—a marker of generalized atherosclerosis affecting all the major blood vessels.

› When atherosclerosis affects some of the arteries to the back, we find an increased risk of degenerative and herniated disk disease.

The common cause

As we have seen, so many of the chronic diseases begin with the interconnected and compounding effects of generalized low-level inflammation, oxidative stress and atherosclerosis. The many specific diseases have different specific names—some well known, many less so—but this bodily process underlies and contributes to all lifestyle diseases, together the cause of the majority of death and disease in our world today.

It is an insidious and progressive disease process—and is directly linked to lifestyle. This presents a sobering challenge, but it's also an exciting possibility. With better education, better understanding and better choices, the most serious diseases in our society today can be reduced and, as has been demonstrated by medical practitioners such as Dr Caldwell Esselstyn, have the potential to be reversed. This is the opportunity offered by lifestyle medicine.

The lifestyle prescription

There are many lifestyle factors that are causal for disease. Poor nutrition, overfeeding, stress, inadequate rest or sleep, inadequate sunshine, irregular or no exercise, toxicity and pollutants—including smoking and alcohol—and the quality of our relationships all have a significant impact on health. By looking at whole-person health as a jigsaw puzzle, with all the pieces interconnected and working together, lifestyle medicine considers the total sum of life events to understand "story" of disease in any individual. It is free of side-effects and is an approach to health care that is within our reach and our abilities. It is a way to simplify life, so we are able to achieve our health and life potentials. Unsurprisingly, the lifestyle medicine prescription looks a lot like that summarized simply by A J Jacobs—"Eat less, move more, relax."

Lifestyle medicine is an approach to health care that is within our reach and our abilities.

› Diet as "medicine"

In their exploration of diet and chronic disease in Chinese population groups published in peer-reviewed medical journals, Dr Campbell and his co-researchers found many links between various food groups and disease conditions that have documented the importance of diet and nutrition as risk factors for disease. His research shows: "People who ate the most animal-based foods got the most chronic disease. Even relatively small intakes of animal-based food were associated with adverse effects. People who ate the most plant-based foods were the healthiest and tended to avoid chronic disease."[12]

The findings of this massive study were remarkable and highlighted the health implications of animal and plant-based nutrients and their differences. The study also drew conclusions about fat, fiber and cholesterol and confirmed there were many links to degenerative diseases such as cancer, heart disease and diabetes. In a practical way, these results underscored the need for dietary interventions for disease management, and the importance of a lifestyle medicine approach. The words of Hippocrates, the father of medicine, remain wise advice: "Let your food be your medicine and your medicine your food."

Hippocrates: "Let your food be your medicine and your medicine your food."

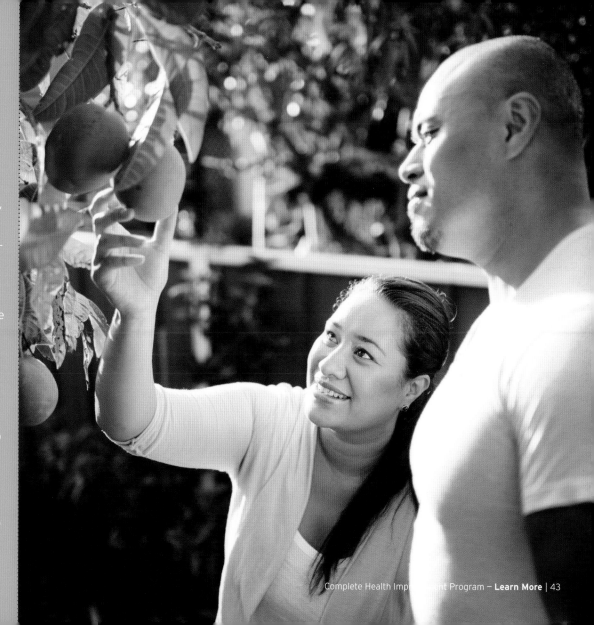

DEFINING "DIET"

The word "diet" can have different connotations. While not its original definition, the word is often taken to mean a structured or restrictive eating plan followed for the purpose of losing weight. But "diet" can also simply mean the kinds of foods a person or community habitually eats. A good example of this second definition is when researchers refer to the "Mediterranean diet," simply a way of describing the kinds of foods a certain community traditionally eats. Another way of explaining this difference in definition could be to say that, while not everyone is dieting, everyone has a diet. Throughout CHIP, you will see and hear a number of references to plant-based diets and the optimal diet. Rather than a restrictive or structured plan, these are simply our way of describing the kinds of eating habits that can contribute to optimal health.

A daily walk outdoors is an enjoyable way to promote optimal health and can be "prescribed" as part of a total disease treatment plan.

› A prescription for exercise

Regular exercise is an important part of a healthy lifestyle and reduces inflammation.[13] A daily walk outdoors is an enjoyable way to promote optimal health and can be "prescribed" as part of a total disease treatment plan. Regular exercise helps the body regulate many vital functions, improves toxin elimination and is a known mood enhancer. Being active, which includes planned exercise and the incidental activity we do as part of everyday life, such as washing the car, walking to the bus stop or playing with a pet, has been shown in countless studies to support healthy aging and a longer life.

› Social and economic factors

Our lifestyles are impacted on by many social, economic and general factors such as where we live, how we live, what support networks we have around us and our values, attitudes and cultural influences. Lifestyle medicine takes into account all these influences and choices on health and wellbeing, looking at these factors as both causal factors and treatment options.

› Stress and mind-body medicine

Many studies show us the way that stress impacts on the body. Stress has oxidizing and inflammatory effects that precede diseases such as cancer and cardiovascular disease. Increasing stress levels have been a by-product of modern living—we work harder, relax less and have much more complex lifestyles than are truly good for us. When stressed, we are also more likely to make poor food choices and exercise less often, so stress often has a compounding effect on other lifestyle factors. Understanding how the mind and body work together for optimal health can provide important insights into our motivation to change.

KEY POINTS

> Most chronic lifestyle diseases have a common cause in chronic low-level inflammation linked to oxidative stress.

> Atherosclerosis, heart disease and many other conditions develop when bad cholesterol is oxidized and builds up as plaque in the blood vessels, restricting and eventually blocking the circulation of blood.

> Undoing this common cause, most lifestyle diseases can be prevented and sometimes potentially reversed by positive lifestyle choices, including the optimal plant-based diet and active lifestyle.

Chapter Three References

1   Jacobs, A J (2012), *Drop Dead Healthy: One Man's Humble Quest for Bodily Perfection,* Simon & Schuster, page 245, emphasis supplied.

2   Egger, G and J Dixon (2010), "Inflammatory effects of nutritional stimuli: further support for the need for a big picture approach to tackling obesity and chronic disease," *Obesity Review,* Vol 11 No 2, pages 137–49.

3   Cosentino, F and G E Assenza (2004), "Diabetes and inflammation," *Herz.* Vol 29 No 8, pages 749–59.

4   Lamon, B D and D P Hajjar (2008), "Inflammation at the molecular interface of atherogenesis: an anthropological journey," *American Journal of Pathology,* Vol 173 No 5, pages 1253–64.

5   Akiyama, H, et al (2000), "Inflammation and Alzheimer's disease," *Neurobiology and Aging,* Vol 21 No 3, pages 383–421.

6   Kondo, T, M Hirose, and K Kageyama (2009), "Roles of oxidative stress and redox regulation in atherosclerosis," *Journal of Atherosclerosis and Thrombosis,* Vol 16 No 5, pages 532–8.

7   "General findings of the International Atherosclerosis Project" (1968), *Laboratory Investigation,* Vol 18 No 5, pages 498–502.

8   Enos, W F, R H Holmes, and J Beyer (1953), "Coronary disease among United States soldiers killed in action in Korea; preliminary report," *Journal of the American Medical Association,* Vol 152 No 12, pages 1090–3.

9   Traub, O, and R Van Bibber (1995), "Role of nitric oxide in insulin-dependent diabetes mellitus-related vascular complications," *Western Journal of Medicine,* Vol 162 No 5, page 439–45; Shimokawa, H (1999), "Primary endothelial dysfunction: atherosclerosis," *Journal of Molecular and Cellular Cardiology,* Vol 31 No 1, pages 23–37.

10   Stamler, J (1978), "George Lyman Duff Memorial Lecture: Lifestyles, major risk factors, proof and public policy," *Circulation,* Vol 58, pages 3–19.

11   Forrester, J S and P K Shah (1997), "Lipid lowering versus revascularization: an idea whose time (for testing) has come," *Circulation,* Vol 96 No 4, page 1360–2.

12   Campbell, T C, B Parpia, and J Chen (1998), "Diet, lifestyle, and the etiology of coronary artery disease: the Cornell China study," *American Journal of Cardiology,* Vol 82 No 10B, pages 18T–21T.

13   Strohacker, K and B K McFarlin (2010), "Influence of obesity, physical inactivity, and weight cycling on chronic inflammation," *Frontiers in Bioscience* (Elite Ed), Vol 2, pages 98–104.

The Optimal Diet

One of the most important lifestyle influences is diet and nutrition. Poor choices can increase disease risks, while the best dietary choices can protect against and potentially reverse chronic disease. A whole-food, plant-based, low-fat, high-fiber diet can change your life and health.

Chapter Four offers an eating plan that allows you to eat as much as you like, while losing weight, in contrast to the common notions of "diets." It comes down to what you eat, not how much.

Chapter Five explains the importance and benefits of fiber in a plant-based eating plan.

Chapter Six explores heart disease—the world's number-one killer. This chapter identifies two of the biggest risks in cholesterol and high blood pressure, and how our lifestyle choices can counteract these common risks.

Chapter Seven discusses the growing epidemic of type 2 diabetes, its impact on the body and how it might be beaten.

Chapter Eight shares eight recommendations from the World Cancer Research Fund, bringing together the best research on reducing the risks of developing cancer.

Chapter Nine addresses some of the most significant myths in relation to plant-based eating. Amid all the research, reports and folk wisdom, advice on diet and nutrition is littered with myths and misinformation, so here are some facts to guide your choices.

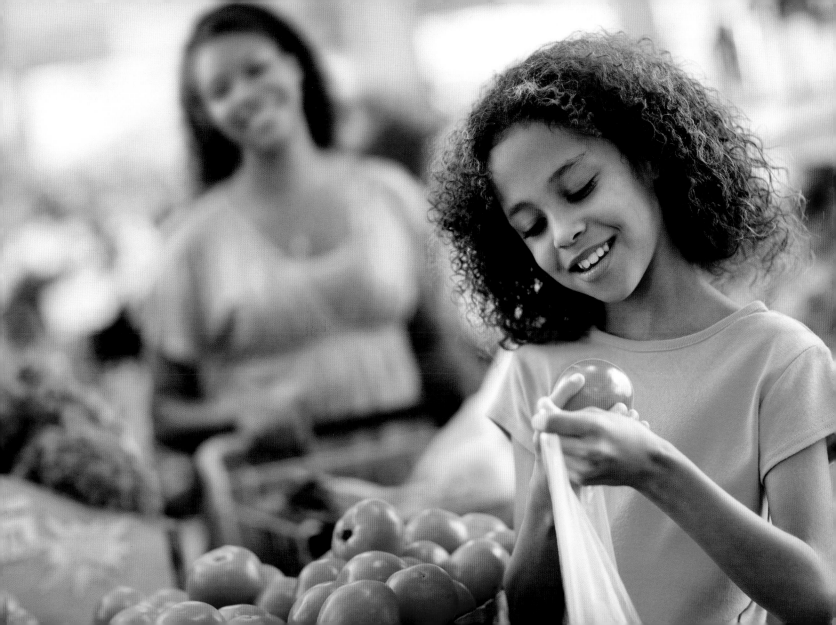

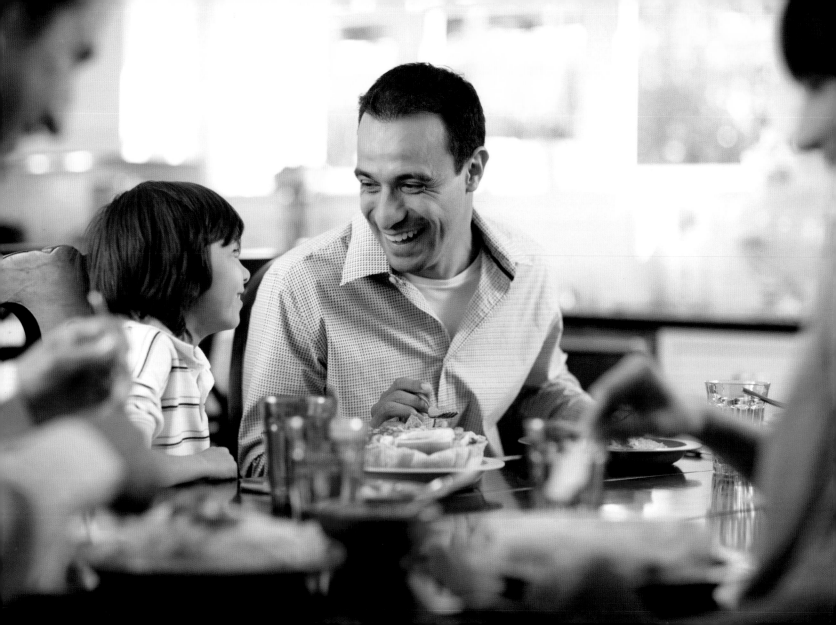

Chapter 4

Eat More, Weigh Less

It sounds like a myth—the ability to eat more and lose weight. But using a couple of simple principles, it is possible, because not all foods are equal when it comes to helping us to feel full.

We're all probably familiar with more than a few strange diets. There are books in your local book store or advice on countless websites that include instructions for a soup diet or a diet where you only eat one fruit for two meals a day or something similar. But the truth is they don't work long term—which means they don't work.

We gain benefits to our health by maintaining a healthy weight long term. These strange diets don't work because they are not sustainable, they're too restrictive and can even be seriously deficient in what a healthy body needs.

Most of us are also familiar with more "normal" dieting techniques, such as calorie restriction or counting calories. But the truth is calorie restriction and calorie counting can also be difficult to maintain over the long term. They can be complicated, restrictive and can leave you feeling hungry, which is not a recipe for success.

The key to maintaining a healthy weight is balancing the energy we consume with the energy we use up through the day. So the key to maintaining a healthy weight is understanding energy in foods.

The key to maintaining a healthy weight is understanding energy in foods, which foods can make you feel fuller while naturally containing less energy.

What is energy?

The food we eat provides the energy necessary for our body to function. Energy is found in fats, proteins, carbohydrates—including starches and sugars—and alcohol. The body uses energy from food for a variety of purposes, including metabolic processes, physiological functions, muscular activity, heat production, growth and synthesis of new tissue. Energy to the body is what fuel is to a car. Without the energy we get from food we would have no fuel.

Fats, protein, carbohydrates and alcohol are all substances the body can digest and get energy from. While each is a source of energy to the body, they contain different amounts of energy. Carbohydrates and protein each contain the least energy per gram, at about 4 Calories per gram. By contrast, fat and alcohol are much more energy dense, containing 9 Calories and 7 Calories per gram, respectively. What this means is that per gram, these contain much more energy and can be easier to overeat.

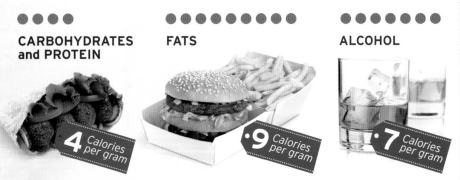

CARBOHYDRATES and PROTEIN
4 Calories per gram

FATS
·9 Calories per gram

ALCOHOL
·7 Calories per gram

Kilojoules and calories[1]

The basic unit of energy is the calorie (imperial—Cal) or the joule (metric—J), commonly expressed as kilojoule (1000 joules—kJ). These units are also used to measure the energy our bodies derive from food eaten and the energy we expend in body processes and activity.

To obtain the equivalent value in calories, divide the kilojoules by 4.18; if converting from calories, multiply by 4.18 to obtain the energy in kilojoules.

For example

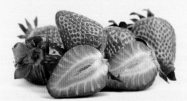

one cup of strawberries contains 120kJ, so 120 divided by 4.18 = 29 calories.

When reading product labels or other food information using an unfamiliar measurement, a simple method is to multiply or divide by 4 to give an approximate conversion.

It's all about balance

If you think about the energy we eat like fuel to a car, there is one key difference. If you try to fill a car with too much fuel, it will simply spill out the top of the fuel tank and make an unpleasant mess on your shoes. You can only put a certain amount of fuel in and after that point you have to stop.

But our bodies aren't like this. They're always looking for ways to protect us against unexpected dangers. So if you eat too much energy, your body will store it as fat in case you run out of food for an extended period of time and need to call on this reserve.

The problem with this—if you can call it a problem—arises when food continues to be readily available and we continue to over-consume. Our bodies simply keep storing more and more. So we need to make sure we balance the amount of energy we are eating with the amount we are using each day. If we eat more than we use, it will lead to weight gain; if we eat less than we use, it will lead to weight loss.

Fundamentally, strategies like calorie counting are based on this fact of energy in and energy out. But strategies like this can be hard to maintain because it's difficult to know the energy content of every food you eat in a day. This adds another level of difficulty to the process of weight loss, something already difficult enough.

On top of this, just because a food contains a certain number or calories or kilojoules, doesn't necessarily mean it's going to fill you up and keep you from feeling hungry. If we eat a diet packed with processed foods, often with large portion sizes, this can be exceptionally challenging.

But there is a solution! If we select foods lower in energy and naturally filling, and we stop eating when we are full, it greatly simplifies the sums of energy in and energy out. This is why whole plant foods play such an important role in maintaining a healthy weight the simple way.

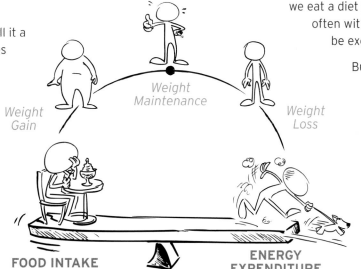

Weight
Maintenance

Weight
Gain

Weight
Loss

FOOD INTAKE

**ENERGY
EXPENDITURE**

What is a healthy weight?

People come in a range of shapes and sizes. While there is no "ideal" body shape, it is important to ensure your height and weight are in proportion, and that you are not carrying too much weight around your waist.

The Body Mass Index (BMI) can be used as a guide to gauge your ideal weight range.[2] A BMI between 18.5 and 25 is considered within a healthy range. If you are above or below this range, your risk of developing health problems is increased. These health problems can include heart disease, type 2 diabetes, gallstones, high blood pressure and certain types of cancer.[3]

However, BMI does have some limitations. For example, BMI does not necessarily reflect body fat distribution and does not necessarily apply to different population groups. It also doesn't apply to infants or children.

How to calculate Body Mass Index

$$BMI = \frac{Weight \text{ (pounds)}}{Height^2 \text{ (inches)}} \times 703 = \frac{Weight \text{ (kilograms)}}{Height^2 \text{ (metres)}}$$

Healthy Weight Tables

Of the various ways of defining ideal weights, the actuarial tables of the Metropolitan Life Insurance Company have also been recognized as helpful. These tables are gender specific and also take into account individual difference in build, being based on height and bone size.[4]

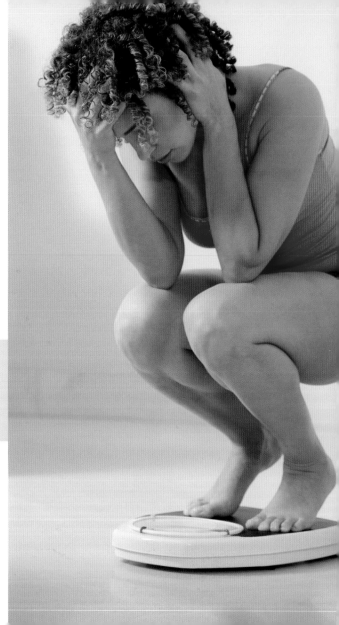

Ideal weights for adults by body frame

Metropolitan Life Insurance Height/Weight Table (1959)

MEN				WOMEN			
HEIGHT (No Shoes)	**SMALL FRAME**	**MEDIUM FRAME**	**LARGE FRAME**	**HEIGHT** (No Shoes)	**SMALL FRAME**	**MEDIUM FRAME**	**LARGE FRAME**
5'2" (157 cm)	115-123 lbs (52-56 kg)	121-133 lbs (55-60 kg)	129-144 lbs (59-65 kg)	4'10" (147 cm)	96-104 lbs (44-47 kg)	101-113 lbs (46-51 kg)	109-125 lbs (49-57 kg)
5'4" (162 cm)	121-129 lbs (55-59 kg)	127-139 lbs (58-63 kg)	135-152 lbs (61-69 kg)	5'0" (152 cm)	102-110 lbs (46-50 kg)	107-119 lbs (49-54 kg)	115-131 lbs (52-59 kg)
5'6" (167 cm)	128-137 lbs (58-62 kg)	134-147 lbs (61-67 kg)	142-161 lbs (64-73 kg)	5'2" (157 cm)	108-116 lbs (49-53 kg)	113-126 lbs (51-57 kg)	121-138 lbs (55-63 kg)
5'8" (173 cm)	136-145 lbs (62-66 kg)	142-156 lbs (64-71 kg)	151-170 lbs (68-77 kg)	5'4" (162 cm)	114-123 lbs (52-56 kg)	120-135 lbs (54-61 kg)	129-146 lbs (59-66 kg)
5'10" (178 cm)	144-154 lbs (65-70 kg)	150-165 lbs (68-75 kg)	159-179 lbs (72-81 kg)	5'6" (167 cm)	122-131 lbs (55-59 kg)	128-143 lbs (58-65 kg)	137-154 lbs (62-70 kg)
6'0" (183 cm)	152-162 lbs (69-73 kg)	158-175 lbs (72-79 kg)	168-189 lbs (76-86 kg)	5'8" (173 cm)	130-140 lbs (59-64 kg)	136-151 lbs (62-68 kg)	145-163 lbs (66-74 kg)
6'2" (188 cm)	160-171 lbs (73-78 kg)	167-185 lbs (76-84 kg)	178-199 lbs (81-90 kg)	5'10" (178 cm)	138-148 lbs (63-67 kg)	144-159 lbs (65-72 kg)	153-173 lbs (69-78 kg)
6'4" (193 cm)	168-179 lbs (76-82 kg)	177-195 lbs (80-88 kg)	187-209 lbs (85-95 kg)	6'0" (183 cm)	148-158 lbs (67-72 kg)	154-169 lbs (70-77 kg)	163-183 lbs (74-83 kg)

Weight includes one pound (450 grams) for ordinary indoor clothing.

How to calculate frame size

Although most people have a pretty good idea of their frame size, wrist–and sometimes ankle–measurements provide a more reliable method.

WOMEN

Small-boned: a wrist measurement of 5.25 inches (13 cm) or less.

Medium-boned: between 5.25 to 6 inches (15 cm).

Large-boned: more than 6 inches.

MEN

Small-boned Anything less than 6 inches (15 cm)

Large-boned: anything more than 7 inches (17.5 cm)

Waist measurement

Another simple way to assess your risk of suffering from a chronic disease is to measure your waist circumference.

To do this, measure halfway between your lowest rib and your hipbone, roughly in line with your belly button. Breathe out normally and make sure the tape is snug without compressing the skin.[5]

WOMEN WAIST MEASUREMENT	RISK OF CHRONIC DISEASE	MEN WAIST MEASUREMENT
Less than or equal to 31.5 inches (80 cm)	Low	Less than or equal to 37 inches (94 cm)
31.5 to 34.5 inches (81 to 88 cm)	Increased	37 to 40 inches (95 to 102 cm)
More than 34.5 inches (88 cm)	Greatly Increased	More than 40 inches (102 cm)

Energy in

All foods supply energy, by providing a source of protein, carbohydrate, fat or alcohol. Most foods contain a combination of these energy sources. But some foods have much higher levels of one or another kind of energy. For example:

> **Foods high in carbohydrate:** breads, cereals, grains (pasta, rice, millet, buckwheat, barley), potato, corn, peas, baked beans, fruit, milk and yoghurt.

> **Foods high in protein:** nuts, eggs, legumes, soy foods (soy milk, soy yoghurt, tofu, soya beans), milk, yoghurt, meat, chicken, fish.

> **Foods high in fat:** fried foods, pastries, cakes, cookies, fatty meats, cheese, avocado, nuts and seeds, oils, margarine, butter, cream.

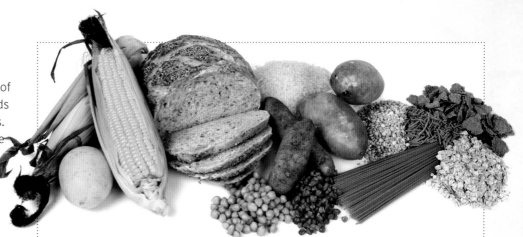

Carbohydrate–THE ULTIMATE FUEL

Health, vitality and energy come from eating a varied, nutritious diet that includes carbohydrates. Carbohydrates are one of the four nutrients in food. They are an ideal source of energy for the body, and particularly important to fuel the brain, as well as power our muscles during exercise.[6]

Sugars are found in carbohydrate foods. They may be naturally occurring or added to food. Foods that have naturally occurring sugars include milk, fruit, and even vegetables and legumes. Sugar can also be refined and this sugar is added to foods or drink such as cakes, cookies and soda/soft drink.

Many people mistakenly think carbohydrates are fattening. This may be true if the carbohydrate comes from foods high in refined simple sugars found in chocolate bars, ice cream and other processed foods. However, if the carbohydrate comes from unrefined natural forms, including whole grains, vegetables or legumes, this is not the case.

The secret to a healthy weight

Energy density is your key to eating more and losing weight. Energy density describes the amount of energy—measured in calories or kilojoules—present in a particular weight of food. Foods with a low energy density provide fewer calories per gram than foods with a higher energy density. This means a person can consume a large portion of low energy-dense food for the same amount of calories as a small portion of high energy-dense food.[7]

Foods with a high energy density include those that are refined and processed. What tends to happen is the water and fiber are removed, so they have less bulk and energy density goes up. Then refined sugars and fats are also often added, making the energy density go up even further.[8]

Low energy-dense foods include whole fruit, whole vegetables and whole grains. Foods with a lower energy density tend to have high water content and lots of fiber. Fiber and water take up space, adding volume and weight to food without adding calories. Plant-based foods (wholefoods) are naturally low in fat, with a few exceptions—such as avocado, nuts and seeds—which should be consumed in moderation. Having a whole-food, plant-based diet can be a great way of losing weight and still enjoying a satisfied feeling during and after a meal.[9]

Studies have shown that eating low energy-dense foods, such as salads or vegetable soup, before the main meal makes people eat less at the main meal and fewer calories in general. Although we do not yet understand all of the mechanisms involved, these foods have high water content—which has weight but contains no calories—and fiber content, so cause you to feel fuller, which leads to eating less energy without you even being aware of it. If you eat foods that are naturally high in water and fiber, you really can eat more and lose weight.

Foods with a lower energy density tend to have high water content and lots of fiber.

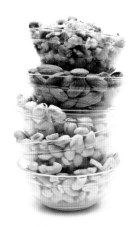

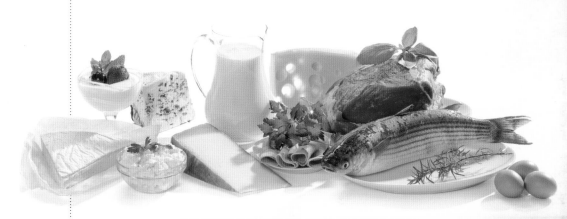

WHAT ABOUT NUTS?

Nuts are a great plant food, being a source of protein, fiber, and some vitamins and minerals. However, nuts are high in fat and even though this is mostly unsaturated fat, this still makes nuts an energy dense food. This does not mean nuts are inherently fattening, but it does mean it can be easier to over-eat nuts compared to low-fat, fiber-rich plant foods, such as vegetables, fruits and wholegrain cereals. As part of an optimal diet, CHIP recommends that nuts be consumed in moderation.

WHERE DO MEAT AND DAIRY FIT?

Meat and dairy products are energy-dense foods. They can be high in fat, while containing no fiber. As part of an optimal diet, CHIP recommends avoiding meat and dairy products, for this and a variety of other reasons. If you choose to include meat and dairy products in your diet, try to think of them more as a condiment, rather than the center of the meal. By doing this and packing meals with good amounts of vegetables and wholegrain cereals, you can keep the energy density of meals down and your weight in a healthy range. If you choose to avoid all animal foods, including dairy, make sure you are getting vitamin B12 regularly from fortified plant foods. Fortified non-dairy milks, such as soy milk, can be a useful source of vitamin B12.

Energy density and satiety

Satiety is the feeling of fullness or satisfaction after a meal. You might be surprised to learn that satiety is not dependent on how much energy a food contains, but if you think about a few examples, it becomes pretty obvious.

Think about one slice of carrot cake and a bowl of 16 carrots. Which one do you think would fill you up more? It's obvious: the 16 carrots are much more filling than the slice of carrot cake— but they have the same energy content!

So how can they get the energy of 16 carrots into one slice of carrot cake? To make a carrot cake, we don't use 16 carrots. Instead we add a number of processed ingredients with high energy densities to the low energy dense carrot, turning it from a health food into a high-energy choice. Refined fats, sugars and flours—all with the fiber and bulk from their original sources removed— can quickly increase the energy density of a food without significantly increasing its ability to help you feel full after a meal.

The extent to which a food fills you depends on a number of things, including its water and fiber content, because water and fiber together form bulk. And bulk is an important contributor of feeling full.[10]

Most diets limit the amount of food you're allowed to eat, but this stimulates hunger. It can be difficult to defeat hunger with willpower, as hunger is a powerful innate survival mechanism. There is an easier way to defeat hunger: eat whole plant foods that maximize satiety.[11]

Satiety and hunger control are important for long-term satisfaction and the ability to stick to healthy eating. Eating low energy-dense foods helps control hunger and maintains a feeling of satiety, which is key to maintaining a healthy weight.[12]

Following these simple principles means you really can eat more but weigh less.

There is a much easier way to defeat hunger: eat whole plant foods that maximize satiety.

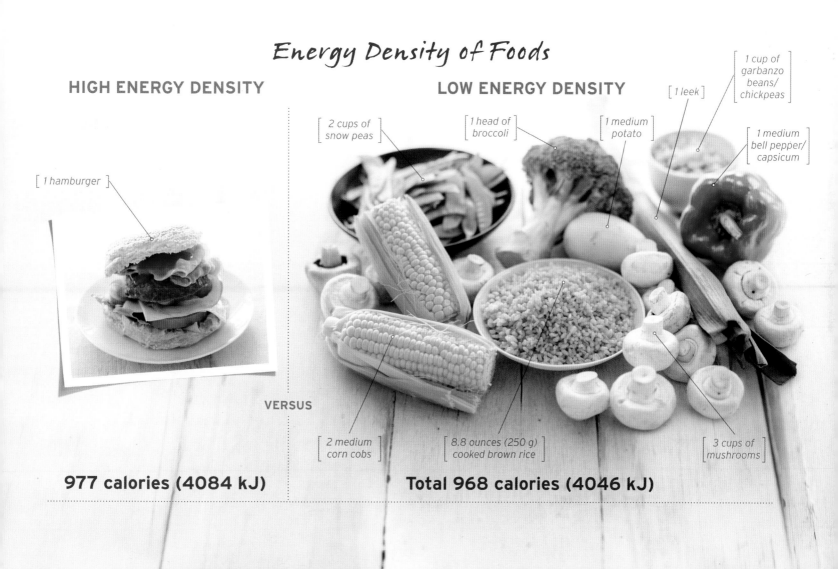

Energy Density of Foods

HIGH ENERGY DENSITY

[1 hamburger]

977 calories (4084 kJ)

VERSUS

LOW ENERGY DENSITY

[2 cups of snow peas]

[1 head of broccoli]

[1 medium potato]

[1 leek]

[1 cup of garbanzo beans/ chickpeas]

[1 medium bell pepper/ capsicum]

[2 medium corn cobs]

[8.8 ounces (250 g) cooked brown rice]

[3 cups of mushrooms]

Total 968 calories (4046 kJ)

Energy Density of Foods

HIGH ENERGY DENSITY

LOW ENERGY DENSITY

CARROT CAKE WITH ICING
1 slice, 5.3 ounces
(150 grams)

503
calories
(2103 kJ)

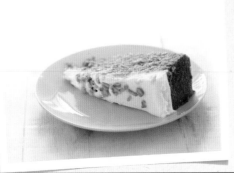

VERSUS

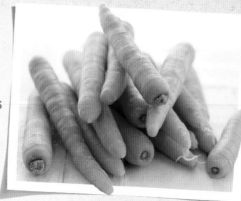

16 CARROTS
3.5 pounds
(1570 grams)

503
calories
(2103 kJ)

5 CHOC CHIP COOKIES
2.1 ounces
(60 grams)

300
calories
(1254 kJ)

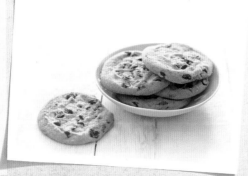

VERSUS

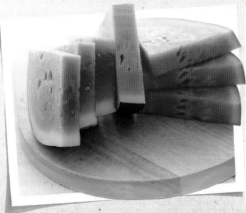

7 THICK SLICES OF WATERMELON
4.5 pounds
(2058 grams)

315
calories
(1317 kJ)

KEY POINTS

> Our body gains necessary energy from the food we eat and naturally stores excess energy as body fat.

> Weight gain or loss is determined by the sum of energy consumed less the energy expended through body processes and activity.

> The energy density of food is a key factor in eating and feeling "full" but not consuming excess energy, so natural unprocessed foods, with high fiber and water content, are important for eating more but weighing less.

Chapter Four References

1   Better Health Channel (2012), "Energy Value," <http://www.betterhealth.vic.gov.au/bhcv2/bhcarticles.nsf/pages/kilojoules_and_calories-explained>.

2   Dietitians Association of Australia, "Body Mass Index," <http://daa.asn.au/for-the-public/smart-eating-for-you/nutrition-a-z/body-mass-index/>.

3   National Heart Blood and Lung Institute, "Assess your weight and health risk," <http://www.nhlbi.nih.gov/health/public/heart/obesity/lose_wt/risk.htm>.

4   "1983 metropolitan height and weight tables," *Statistics Bulletin of the Metropolitan Life Foundation,* Vol 64 No 1, pages 3–9.

5   Australian Government (2003), "How to measure yourself," <http://www.measureup.gov.au/internet/abhi/publishing.nsf/Content/How+do+I+measure+myself-lp#measuring>.

6   Dietitians Association of Australia, "Sugar," <http://daa.asn.au/for-the-public/smart-eating-for-you/nutrition-a-z/sugars/>.

7   Rolls, B J (2009), "The relationship between dietary energy density and energy intake," *Physiology and Behavior,* Vol 97 No 5, pages 609–15.

8   ibid.

9   Rolls, B J, et al (1999), "Water incorporated into a food but not served with a food decreases energy intake in lean women," *American Journal of Clinical Nutrition,* Vol 70 No 4, pages 448–55.

10   Bell, E A, et al (1998), "Energy density of foods affects energy intake in normal-weight women," *American Journal of Clinical Nutrition,* Vol 67 No 3, pages 412–20.

11   Carmagnola, S, et al (2005), "Mechanoreceptors of the Proximal Stomach and Perception of Gastric Distension," *American Journal of Gastroenterology,* Vol 100 No 8, pages 1704–10.

12   Department of Health and Human Services USA, "Low-Energy-Dense foods and Weight Management: Cutting Calories While Controlling Hunger," <http://www.cdc.gov/nccdphp/dnpa/nutrition/pdf/r2p_energy_density.pdf>.

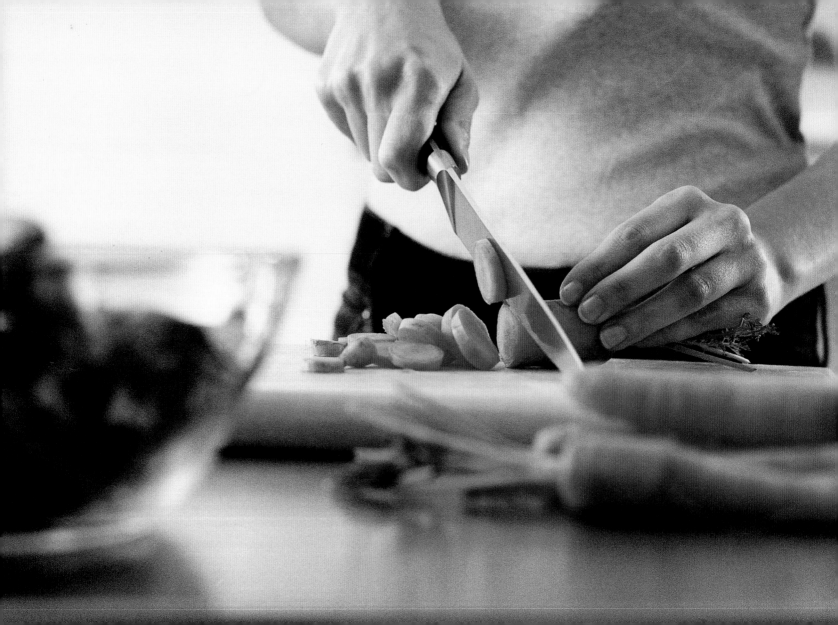

Chapter Five

Fiber, Your New Best Friend

One of the keys to maintaining healthy lifestyle choices is a good support group. Like-minded and committed friends can help motivate us, support us through our difficult times and keep us on track. But, if there were ever a nutritional version of a best friend, it would be fiber. While making new friends isn't always easy, putting in the time to get to know fiber is worthwhile. It's a great friend to have. When a lot of us think of fiber, we probably think of keeping "regular," which can be a great benefit of fiber. But fiber has so much more to offer.

Fiber can be there at every meal to help protect you from overeating. Fiber can also be your friend when making food choices, helping point out which foods are nutritious and low in calories. It can even help decrease your risk of a range of chronic diseases!

You can never have too many friends, so take the time to get to know dietary fiber.

What is dietary fiber?

Dietary fiber is found only in foods of plant origin, such as grains, legumes, vegetables, fruit, nuts and seeds. It is not found in meat, poultry, fish, eggs or dairy products. It is part of a plant that undergoes some digestion in the small intestine, before being transported to the large intestine (colon), where it is further broken down by an army of beneficial bacteria.[1]

Dietary fiber is found only in foods of plant origin.

There are two major types of fiber—insoluble and soluble. Both play an important role in maintaining a healthy digestive system. These different types of fiber perform different roles in the body, so we need enough fiber from a range of foods to maintain good health.[2]

Insoluble fiber includes substances such as cellulose, hemicelluloses and lignin. This type of fiber adds bulk to feces, and helps prevent constipation and associated problems such as hemorrhoids. Insoluble fiber does not dissolve in water, which gives it the ability to draw water into the stools, making them larger, softer and easier to pass. Rich sources of insoluble fiber include wholegrain wheat and wheat bran, rice bran, vegetables, nuts and seeds.

Soluble fiber is found in oats and oat bran, barley, psyllium, flaxseed, beans, lentils, soy beans and fruits. Soluble fiber works by forming a thick gel with water, which is then broken down by good bacteria in the colon, releasing substances that help keep the bowel wall healthy. Research has even shown some types of soluble fiber to be effective in lowering blood cholesterol levels.[3]

Research has even shown some types of soluble fiber to be effective in lowering blood cholesterol levels.

Resistant starch

Resistant starch is not traditionally thought of as fiber, but it acts in a similar way and is often classified as fiber. Resistant starch is the part of starchy food—approximately 10 per cent—that resists normal digestion, and therefore has many of the same functions as soluble and insoluble fiber.

This starch is found in many unprocessed cereals and grains like pearl barley and brown rice, and is sometimes added to processed grain foods like bread and breakfast cereals. It is also found in legumes, like lentils and baked beans, and cooled cooked potato, rice and pasta.

Bacteria in the large bowel ferment and change the resistant starch into short-chain fatty acids, which are important to bowel health and may protect against cancer. These fatty acids are also absorbed into the bloodstream and may play a role in lowering blood cholesterol levels.[4]

Good bacteria

You might have heard the term "probiotics." These are the good bacteria that produce the fuel that gut cells thrive on. There are trillions of bacteria in the gastrointestinal tract. In most people, the correct balance of good bacteria is maintained in the digestive system by eating a variety of health foods.[5] Probiotic products can be found in certain foods such as some yoghurts and fermented milk drinks, as well as supplements that can come in the form of dried powders and capsules.

If you imagine probiotics as the flowers in a garden, prebiotics are the soil they can thrive in. They're food for the good bacteria. Growth of beneficial bacteria is supported by fiber-rich foods, including whole grains, beans and legumes, fruits and vegetables, which naturally contain prebiotics.[6]

We want to nourish the good bacteria with plenty of fiber. Not only do they provide fuel for the gut cells, they also fight bad bacteria and produce some vitamins! What's more, this healthy balance of good bacteria and healthy gut cells also helps stimulate normal bowel movements, nutrient absorption and energy production.[7]

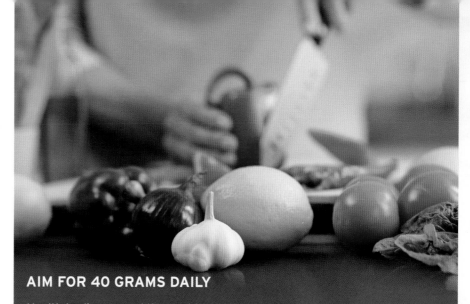

AIM FOR 40 GRAMS DAILY

Health bodies around the world recommend a variety of minimum target ranges of dietary fiber. We recommend aiming to eat 40 grams or more of fiber per day. The reason for this is the many health benefits a high-fiber diet can provide, which extend beyond gut health to the areas such as satiety and weight control and is helpful for the control of blood sugar levels. Fiber is not thought to have an upper limit for consumption and there is no evidence that too much fiber might be unhealthy.[8]

While 40 grams may sound like a large amount of fiber, following a whole-food, plant-based diet can make it easy to consume this much and more on a daily basis. Fiber can also be thought of as a marker of a healthy whole food, as whole foods that are naturally high in fiber tend to be packed full of a range of important nutrients, while often being low in caloric energy. Check out the table of high-fiber foods on the next two pages to see how much fiber you are consuming each day.

Foods Dietary Fiber (measured in grams)

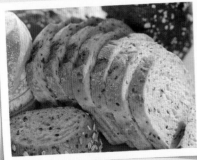

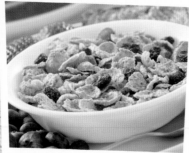

RICE AND PASTA (cooked)

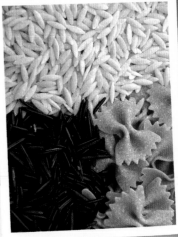

WHOLE WHEAT PASTA (½ cup)	6.0
BROWN RICE (½ cup)	1.5
WHITE PASTA (½ cup)	1.5
WHITE RICE (½ cup)	0.5

LEGUMES (cooked)

BAKED BEANS canned (½ cup)	8.0
MUNG BEANS (½ cup)	7.5
LENTILS (½ cup)	7.5
SOYA BEANS (½ cup)	6.1
MIXED BEANS canned (½ cup)	6.0
RED KIDNEY BEANS (½ cup)	6.0
LIMA/HARICOT BEANS (½ cup)	6.0
BUTTER BEANS (½ cup)	5.0
CHICK PEAS (½ cup)	4.3

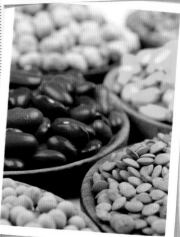

BREAD

MIXED GRAIN (2 slices)	5.0
SOY & LINSEED (2 slices)	5.0
WHOLE WHEAT (2 slices)	4.0
BROWN (2 slices)	3.0
FIBER-INCREASED WHITE (2 slices)	3.0
FRUIT LOAF (2 slices)	2.0
WHITE (2 slices)	2.0

BREAKFAST CEREAL

BRAN (½ cup)	9.5
WHEAT BRAN (2 tablespoons)	5.5
RICE BRAN (2 tablespoons)	4.0
WHEAT BISCUITS (2 biscuits)	4.0
ROLLED OATS cooked (1 cup)	3.5
MUESLI (½ cup)	3.5
OAT BRAN (2 tablespoons)	3.0

VEGETABLES

BRUSSELS SPROUTS cooked *(5 average)*	5.5
GREEN PEAS cooked *(½ cup)*	5.5
CARROT raw *(1 medium)*	4.5
BEETROOT *(1 medium)*	4.0
SWEET CORN *(small cob)*	4.0
BROCCOLI cooked *(1 medium stalk)*	3.0
SPINACH *(½ cup)*	3.0
TOMATOES *(1 medium)*	2.5
CABBAGE cooked *(½ cup)*	2.0
CAULIFLOWER *(1 floweret)*	2.0
POTATOES boiled in skin *(1 medium)*	2.0
LETTUCE *(3 leaves)*	1.0

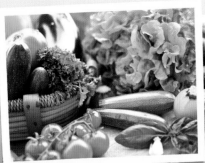
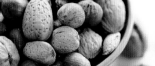

FRUIT

GRAPES *(1 small bunch)*	4.0	**PEAR** *(1 medium)*	6.0
APPLE *(1 medium)*	4.0	**PRUNES** *(6 pitted)*	4.0
BANANA *(1 medium)*	3.0	**PAWPAW (PAPAYA)** *(1 cup diced)*	3.5
KIWI FRUIT *(1 medium)*	3.0	**SULTANAS** *(½ cup)*	3.5
APRICOTS dried *(5 - 6 halves)*	2.5	**STRAWBERRIES** *(1 medium stalk)*	3.0
DATES *(4 pitted)*	3.0	**ORANGE** *(1 medium)*	3.0
BLUEBERRIES *(½ cup)*	1.5	**PASSIONFRUIT** *(1 medium)*	2.5
FRUIT JUICE *(1 cup)*	Trace amounts	**PEACH** *(1 medium)*	2.5
		WATERMELON *(1 cup)*	1.0

NUTS AND SEEDS

PISTACHIOS *(1oz/30g/small handful)*	3.0
SESAME SEEDS *(1oz/30g)*	3.0
SUNFLOWER SEEDS *(1oz/30g)*	3.0
ALMOND *(1oz/30g/small handful)*	2.5
PEANUTS raw *(1oz/30g/small handful)*	2.5
CASHEWS *(1oz/30g/small handful)*	2.0
WALNUTS *(1oz/30g/small handful)*	2.0

OTHER FOODS

MEAT, FISH, CHICKEN, EGGS, CHEESE, MILK, YOGHURT, FATS AND OILS, SWEET BISCUITS, CAKES, SWEETS AND CANDIES, ALCOHOL

Trace amounts

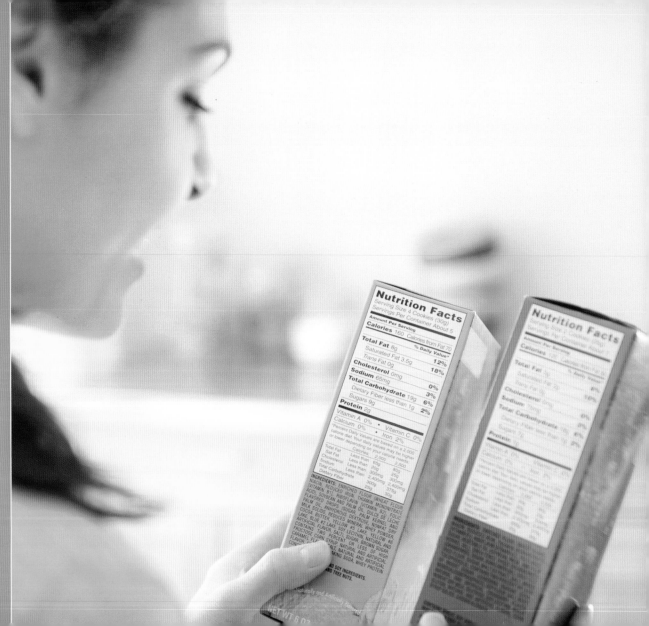

BE LABEL SMART

An optimal way of eating is based around whole, unprocessed plant foods. However, some staple packaged foods, like whole wheat bread, can fit well into a nutritious diet. When choosing packaged foods, read the labels to help you choose foods that contain good amounts of fiber. Claims for fiber differ around the world based on local food-labelling laws, but a useful tip is to aim for foods that contain at least 3 grams of fiber per serving.

The effects of fiber

Besides helping keep the gut nourished and healthy, a high-fiber diet may decrease the risk of a number of specific conditions:[9]

› Constipation

Constipation is the passing of hard, dry bowel motions (stools) that may be infrequent or difficult to pass. The most common causes of constipation include:[10]

Low-fiber diet: As fiber is indigestible, it adds bulk to the feces and makes it easier to push along the digestive tract.

Inadequate fluid intake: Water plumps up the fiber in the feces. Even people who have a high-fiber diet can be constipated if they don't drink enough water.

Low level of exercise: Living a largely sedentary lifestyle and lack of physical activity.

A change in routine: Often seen in shift workers and travellers.

Other factors that may cause constipation include medications, pregnancy, advancing age, illness and delaying toilet trips.

Keys to healthy bowel movements

› Aim to eat at least 40 grams of fiber each day.

› Drink plenty of water each day to help the fiber work properly.

› Get active—at least 30 minutes per day.

› Introduce fiber slowly into your diet to prevent constipation or diarrhea.

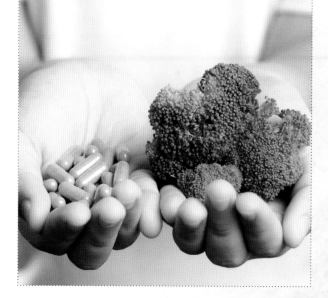

Fiber supplements

Fiber supplements come in a variety of forms, including capsules and powders that can be dissolved into drinks. While they can boost our daily fiber intake, they generally contain only one type of fiber, rather than the wide range of fibers obtained from different foods eaten throughout the day. Aim to get fiber from a wide range of whole foods to gain maximum benefit with minimum fuss.

› Diverticular disease

Diverticulosis occurs when small defects in the muscle of the wall of the large intestine or colon allow small pockets or pouches (diverticula) to form. This happens when the pressure inside the colon increases, in other words, when constipation occurs. Diverticulitis occurs when these abnormal pouches become infected or inflamed. Together, these conditions are called diverticular disease.[11]

Diverticulosis is fairly uncommon for people under the age of 40, with a prevalence of about 4 per cent, but this figure rises to 65 per cent for 65 years or older.[12]

	DIVERTICULOSIS	DIVERTICULITIS
SYMPTOMS	• Abdominal discomfort and bloating • Constipation and diarrhea • Flatulence • Blood in the feces—usually minor, bleeding can sometimes be heavy if a diverticulum gets inflamed or is near a blood vessel • Anemia from repeated bleeding may occur	• Sharp pain, often located at a specific point—for example, in the lower left half of the abdomen • Fever • Distension (bloating) of the abdomen • Nausea and vomiting
TREATMENT *Any dietary changes should be discussed and planned with your physician who can work with you to ensure optimal outcomes.*	• A gradual switch to a diet with increased soluble fiber • Some foods may make symptoms worse or even lead to diverticulitis • Short-term use of fiber supplements	• No eating or drinking—intravenous fluids are given to rest the bowel • Antibiotics and medications • Possible surgery and colostomy

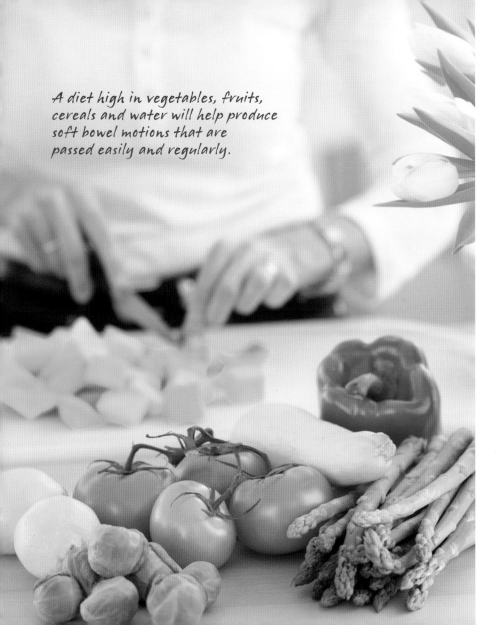

A diet high in vegetables, fruits, cereals and water will help produce soft bowel motions that are passed easily and regularly.

› Hemorrhoids

Hemorrhoids—also known as piles—are varicose veins of the rectum or anus. They are common in middle and later life, often caused by years of chronic constipation.[13]

Bleeding is the most common symptom of hemorrhoids. Most people with internal hemorrhoids notice a smear of bright-red blood on the toilet paper or perhaps streaks of blood in the feces. It is important to see a doctor, because bleeding from the bowel can be caused by other conditions, some of them serious, including bowel cancer.

Both treating and preventing hemorrhoids relies on eliminating constipation, primarily through dietary change. A diet high in vegetables, fruits, cereals and water will help produce soft bowel motions that are passed easily and regularly.

› Colorectal cancer

Also called bowel cancer, colorectal cancer is the third most common cancer worldwide, with around 1.2 million cases documented in 2008.[14] It mostly affects people 50 years of age and older, but it can happen in younger people. In fact, in Australia, which has the highest rates in the world, there has been a 64 per cent increase in the incidence of bowel cancer among 20 to 34 year olds since the mid-1990s.[15] It is a serious disease but if bowel cancer or its precursors (polyps) are diagnosed early, 90 per cent of cases can be treated successfully.[16]

The bowel is the long "tube" that absorbs water and nutrients from food and processes waste products into feces. It includes the small bowel, colon and rectum. Bowel cancer is caused by the uncontrolled growth of abnormal cells forming a tumor within the colon or rectum.

Most bowel cancer develops from small growths called polyps, although not all polyps are cancerous. If polyps are removed, the risk of bowel cancer is reduced. Development of polyps and whether or not they become cancerous depends on a range of factors including genetic, environmental and lifestyle.

RISK FACTORS FOR COLORECTAL CANCER

The causes of bowel cancer are not clearly understood. However, some risk factors make it more likely that a person will develop bowel cancer. These include:[17]

- **Getting older:** Bowel cancer is more common in people older than 50.
- **Genetics:** Two uncommon genetic disorders increase your risk—familial adenomatous polyposis (FAP) or hereditary non-polyposis colorectal cancer (HNPCC).
- **A strong family history of bowel cancer or polyp development.**
- **Inflammatory bowel disease:** Conditions such as ulcerative colitis (inflamed colon lining) or Crohn's disease can increase your risk.
- **Lifestyle choices:** A diet high in red and processed meat, drinking too much alcohol and smoking may increase your risk of developing bowel cancer.
- **Weight:** Being overweight or obese may increase the risk of bowel cancer, particularly for men.

When age is the only standing risk factor for bowel cancer, a colonoscopy is recommended every five to 10 years after the age of 50.[18] If you have other risk factors, you will need to have them more regularly and speak to your doctor about this. The Cancer Council recommends a fecal occult blood test and a sigmoidoscopy every 5 years as screening tests for bowel cancer.

Diet helps

A diet naturally high in fiber helps reduce the risk of developing colorectal cancer. The European Prospective Investigation into Cancer and Nutrition (EPIC) study reported a linear decrease in the risk of colorectal cancer with increasing fiber intake.[19] There may be various reasons this is the case. For instance, adequate fiber may help by preventing constipation, diluting and binding cancer-related toxins in the bowels and reducing the time these toxins are in contact with the bowel wall. Diets naturally high in fiber may also help by supplying other anti-cancer components and fiber helps the body to get rid of free radicals, which can be involved in the development of cancer.[20]

Whichever way fiber-rich eating helps reduce the risk of colorectal cancer, it pays to follow a naturally high-fiber diet with abundant fruit, vegetables and whole grains, while avoiding red and processed meat and alcohol, which are considered to be convincing dietary risk factors for colorectal cancer.[21]

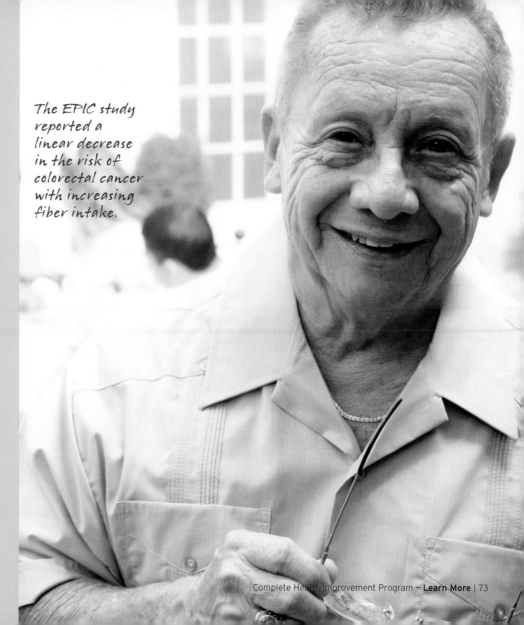

The EPIC study reported a linear decrease in the risk of colorectal cancer with increasing fiber intake.

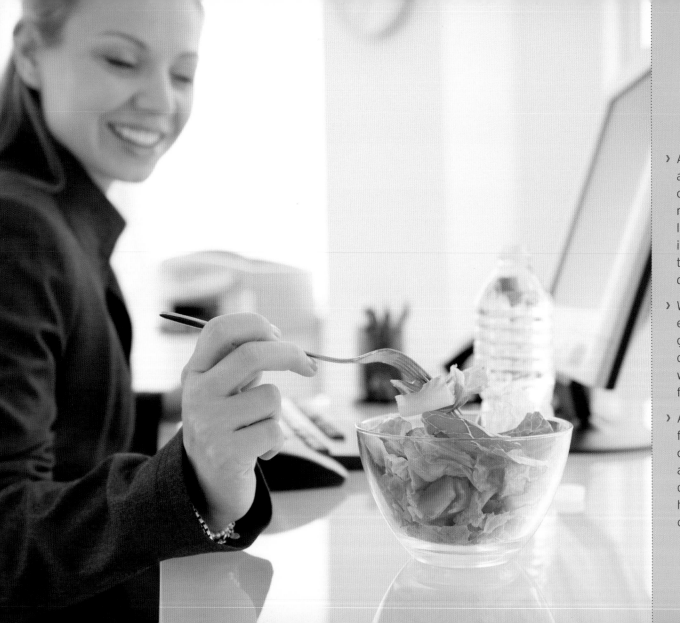

KEY POINTS

› As well as being an important component in eating more and weighing less, dietary fiber is important for the health of our digestive system.

› We should aim to eat at least 40 grams of fiber per day, drawn from a wide variety of plant foods.

› Adequate dietary fiber reduces risks of conditions such as colorectal cancer, diverticular disease, hemorrhoids and constipation.

Chapter Five References

1   Isolauri, E, et al (2002), "Probiotics: A role in the treatment of intestinal infection and inflammation?" GUT: An International Journal of Gastroenterology and Hepatology, Vol 50 Supplement 3, pages III54–9.

2   Anderson, J W, et al (2009), "Health benefits of dietary fiber," Nutrition Reviews, Vol 67 No 4, pages 188–205.

3   Brown, L, et al (1999), "Cholesterol-lowering effects of dietary fiber: a meta-analysis," American Journal of Clinical Nutrition, Vol 69 No 1, pages 30–42.

4   Better Health Channel (2012), "Fibre in food," <http://www.betterhealth.vic. gov.au/bhcv2/bhcarticles.nsf/pages/fibre_in_food>.

5   Aune, D, et al (2011), "Dietary fiber, whole grains, and risk of colorectal cancer: systematic review and dose-response meta-analysis of prospective studies," British Medical Journal, Vol 343, d6617; World Cancer Research Fund/American Institute for Cancer Research (2007), Food, nutrition, physical activity and the prevention of cancer: a global perspective, AICR; Salmeron, J, et al (1997), "Dietary Fiber, Glycemic Load, and Risk of NIDDM in Men," Diabetes Care, Vol 20 No 4, pages 545–50.

6   Aune, et al (2011), op cit; Bingham, S A, et al (2003), "Dietary fiber in food and protection against colorectal cancer in the European Prospective Investigation into Cancer and Nutrition (EPIC): an observational study," Lancet, Vol 361, pages 1496–501; Ferlay, J, et al (2010), "Estimates of worldwide burden of cancer in 2008: GLOBOCAN 2008," International Journal of Cancer, Vol 127, pages 2893–917.

7   Cani, P D, et al (2007), "Selective increases of bifidobacteria in gut microflora improve the high-fat-diet-induced diabetes in mice through a mechanism associated with endotoxemia," Diabetologia, Vol 50 No 11, pages 2374–83; Andromanakos, N, et al (2006), "Constipation of anorectal outlet obstruction: pathophysiology, evaluation and management," Journal of Gastroenterology and Hepatology, Vol 21 No 4, pages 638–46.

8   National Health and Medical Research Council and New Zealand Ministry of Health (2006), "Nutrient Reference Values for Australia and New Zealand Including Recommended Dietary Intakes: Dietary Fibre," NHMRC.

9   Better Health Channel (2012), "Fibre in food," <http://www.betterhealth.vic. gov.au/bhcv2/bhcarticles.nsf/pages/fibre_in_food>.

10 Better Health Channel (2012), "Constipation," <http://www.betterhealth.vic. gov.au/bhcv2/bhcarticles.nsf/pages/Constipation>.

11 Better Health Channel (2012), "Diverticulosis and diverticulitis," <http:// www.betterhealth.vic.gov.au/bhcv2/bhcarticles.nsf/pages/Diverticulosis_ and_diverticulitis?open>.

12 Comparato, G, et al (2007), "Diverticular disease in the elderly," Digestive Diseases, Vol 25 No 2, pages 151–9.

13 Alonso-Coello, P, et al (2006), "Clinical Review: Fiber for the Treatment of Hemorrhoids Complications: A Systematic Review and Meta-Analysis," American Journal of Gastroenterology, Vol 101 No 1, pages 181–8.

14 Ferlay (2010), op cit.

15 Better Health Channel (2012), "Bowel Cancer," <http://www.betterhealth.vic. gov.au/bhcv2/bhcarticles.nsf/pages/bowel_cancer>.

16 Healthy Food Guide (2012), "Bowel Cancer Screening," <http://www. storycentral.com.au/assets/releases/11829/food-bowel-cancer-special- report.pdf>.

17 Australian Goverment Department of Health and Aging (2008), "Familial aspects of bowel cancer: A guide for health professionals."

18 Healthy Food Guide (2012), "Bowel Cancer Screening," <http://www. storycentral.com.au/assets/releases/11829/food-bowel-cancer-special- report.pdf>.

19 Bingham (2003), op cit.

20 Trock, B, et al (1990), "Dietary Fiber, Vegetables, and Colon Cancer: Critical Review and Meta-analyses of the Epidemiologic Evidence," Journal of the National Cancer Institute, Vol 82 No 8, pages 650–61.

21 World Cancer Research Fund/American Institute for Cancer Research (2007), op cit.

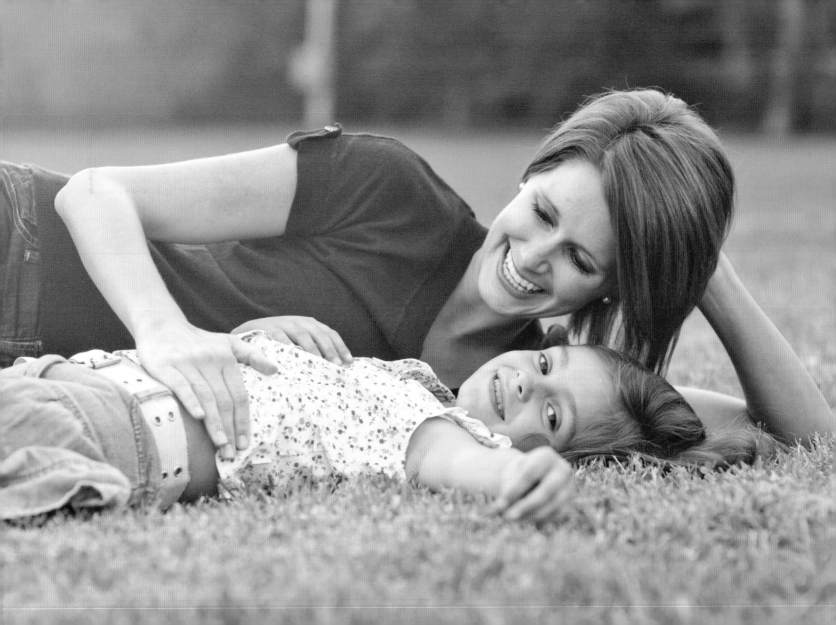

Chapter Six

The Heart of the Matter

The human heart is a miraculous organ. In an average lifetime, it will faithfully beat around 3 billion times, transporting blood, with the oxygen and nutrients it contains, to where they are needed around the body. In simple terms, the heart is a pump, pumping blood through the tens of thousands of miles of our circulatory system.

In some ways, this system is like a water feature or fountain. While everything is working properly, it's a wonder to behold, but if one of any number of things goes wrong with the plumbing, it can slowly lose effectiveness or even suddenly shut off.

When this happens with a fountain, a plumber will check a number of things. The first thing they'll check is if the pump is still working. If it is, the next thing they check is if something is blocking the pipes. Perhaps dirt or leaves have gotten into the plumbing or maybe the water has left mineral deposits that need to be cleaned out.

As complex as the human heart and circulatory system are, they can fall victim to these same simple problems of plumbing. Something can happen to our pump—the heart—or, more commonly, our blood vessels—the pipes—can become clogged or completely blocked.

Cardiovascular disease (CVD) is the term used to describe a range of conditions, including heart attack, stroke and blood vessel diseases. The main cause of CVD is atherosclerosis. As we have seen, this occurs when cholesterol, fat and other substances build up inside the blood vessel walls. The vessels become narrow or even completely

According to the World Health Organization, cardiovascular disease is the world's leading cause of death.

Kinds of Cardiovascular Disease

There are a number of different types of cardiovascular disease but those we will be focusing on in this chapter are

Heart attack
A heart attack happens when there is a sudden blockage to an artery that supplies blood to the heart.

Coronary heart disease
When arteries that supply the heart become clogged, this is known as coronary heart disease. This chronic disease is the most common cause of death in the developed world. It is also a major cause of disability, with many people reporting problems or needing assistance with daily activities.

Cerebrovascular disease (stroke)
Rapid loss of brain function due to disturbance in blood supply to the brain, often leading to varying degrees of loss of mental or physical function.

High blood pressure
High blood pressure—also known as hypertension—is caused by increased pressure in the arteries as the heart pumps blood around the body.

Heart failure
Heart failure occurs when the heart muscle has become too weak to pump blood effectively through the body.

Angina
Angina is chest pain or discomfort caused by insufficient blood flow and oxygen to the muscle of the heart.

block up, so little or no blood can travel through to the brain, heart and other organs.

When the arteries that supply the heart become clogged, this is known as coronary heart disease (CHD), where the heart stops getting all the oxygen it wants to keep functioning efficiently, and this can result in angina or heart attack. When blood supply to the brain is reduced or blocked, this can cause a stroke.[1]

According to the World Health Organization, cardiovascular disease is the world's leading cause of death.[2]

Atherosclerosis re-visited

First, let's re-cap from Chapter 3. Atherosclerosis is a disease in which plaque builds up inside the arteries. This plaque is made up of fat, cholesterol, calcium, and other substances found in the blood. The body naturally produces nitric oxide, which helps keep arteries healthy and flexible, and blood flowing freely. However, when plaque oxidizes on the artery walls, it causes damage that stops this natural process from occurring.[3] This contributes to the build-up of plaque, associated with inflammation, a loss of flexibility and a thickening of the walls of the artery.

Over time, plaque continues to build up, hardening and narrowing the arteries. This limits the flow of oxygen-rich blood to your organs and other parts of your body where they are so vitally needed. Not to be taken lightly, atherosclerosis can lead to heart attack, stroke and even sudden death.[4]

What's more, atherosclerosis is "silent." We cannot feel it developing and the first sign of it can be sudden death! Atherosclerosis is a progressive disease that builds up over many years, even beginning in childhood.[5]

Atherosclerosis is "silent." We cannot feel it developing and the first sign of it can be sudden death!

Cholesterol questions

Everyone has cholesterol. It is a waxy, fat-like substance in our blood and is produced in the liver. It is a part of all animal cells and is essential for many of the body's metabolic processes, including hormone and bile production, and to help the body use vitamin D.

Cholesterol in the diet comes only from foods derived from animals. Plant foods do not contain cholesterol. In fact, many plant foods contain a type of fiber that helps lower cholesterol. However, there's no need to eat foods high in cholesterol as the body is very good at making its own and can make all it needs.[6] Too much cholesterol in the diet can be a key contributor to the formation of arterial plaques.

Cholesterol is carried around in the blood in two key forms:

> **Low density lipoprotein** (LDL) cholesterol is known as "bad cholesterol," because an excess can build up inside the walls of the arteries.

> **High density lipoprotein** (HDL) cholesterol has been referred to as "good cholesterol" and is thought to help remove bad cholesterol from the blood.

What is a healthy blood cholesterol level?

In different parts of the world, cholesterol is measured in either milligram per deciliter (mg/dL)—or millimoles per litre (mmol/L)—of blood. Commonly recommended cholesterol levels to aim for are:[7]

> Less than 210 mg/dL (5.5 mmol/L) total blood cholesterol

> No more than 115 mg/dL (3 mmol/L) for LDL cholesterol

> More than 40 mg/dL (1 mmol/L) for HDL cholesterol

CHIP recognises these recommendations, but believes the research suggests real benefits can be obtained by aiming for lower cholesterol targets,[8] with data showing a further reduction of cardiac risk by achieving levels lower than those commonly recommended.[9]

Because of this, CHIP recommends participants aim for cholesterol levels of:

> **Less than 160 mg/dL (4.2mmol/L) total cholesterol**

> **Less than 90 mg/dL (2.3 mmol/L) for LDL cholesterol**

Remember, we can reduce the risk of developing atherosclerosis by reducing excess LDL cholesterol, as well as by reducing the risk of the LDL cholesterol being oxidized.[10]

Researchers report a 1 to 3 per cent decrease in atherosclerosis risk for every 1 per cent decrease in blood LDL cholesterol.[11] Results from CHIP studies indicate that it is possible to achieve reductions of up to 20 per cent in total cholesterol and LDL cholesterol, usually within four weeks.[12]

Fighting cholesterol

Research suggests that the two key components in the formation of atherosclerotic plaques are cholesterol and oxidation. So it makes sense to try to keep our blood cholesterol levels down and reduce the amount of oxidative stress inside our body. The great news is that diet and activity can play a large role in achieving this.

- To start with, by minimizing our consumption of cholesterol and dietary fats, we can help reduce our risk of excess LDL cholesterol circulating in the blood.

- Key to lowering our LDL cholesterol is to limit the saturated fat and trans fats in our diet.[13] Most of the foods in the list opposite are either processed foods or foods of animal origin. In contrast, a whole food, plant-based diet is naturally low in saturated and trans fats and will reduce the amount of LDL cholesterol in our blood.

- But an eating pattern naturally low in fat—particularly saturated fats and trans fats—and cholesterol can also help reduce the risk of LDL becoming oxidized. A whole foods,

The bad fats[14]

These fats increase blood cholesterol and all should be avoided.

SATURATED FATS	TRANS FATS
› Butter, lard, ghee, copha, cooking margarine, solid frying fats	› Naturally occurring in meat and dairy products from ruminant animals.
› Chocolate and snack foods	› Created in processed oils subject to a process called partial hydrogenation.
› Fatty meats (sausages, salami, processed meats, visible white fat, skin on chicken)	› Trans fats can be present in:
› Full-cream dairy (milk, cheese, yoghurt, ice-cream, cream)	• Deep-fried foods (spring rolls, fried chicken, hot potato chips or fries)
› Palm oils (commonly used in fast foods, biscuits, cakes and pastries)	• Fast-food meals and baked goods (pies, pastries, cakes, cookies, meat pies and buns)
› Coconut oil, coconut milk, coconut cream	

While some cooking oils are better choices than others with regard to heart health, it is important to remember that all cooking oils contain a certain amount of saturated fat. On top of this, they are all equally nutrient-dense.

plant-based diet is also naturally high in potent antioxidants, such as vitamins C and E, and polyphenols, and can also help protect against oxidative stress.[15] Research has also shown a type of soluble fiber called beta-glucans, found in oats and barley, can actively work to help reduce blood cholesterol levels.[16]

How activity helps

Research has shown exercise can be effective in raising the levels of HDL cholesterol circulating in the blood.[17] Adding to this benefit, being active can also increase our antioxidant capacity,[18] meaning exercise can not only increase our levels of good cholesterol, but also works to decrease the risk of LDL cholesterol being oxidized.

Triglycerides count

Triglycerides are another type of fat in the blood. Levels are not as stable as cholesterol levels and, in most cases, they can easily be influenced by diet from one day to the next. However, if higher than 500 mg/dL (5.7 mmol/L), talk to your doctor.

RISKS	TRIGLYCERIDES mg/dL(mmol/L)
Ideal	Less than 150 (1.7)
Elevated	150-199 (1.7-2.2)
High	200-299 (2.3-3.4)
Very High	300-499 (3.5-5.7)
Extremely High	500 plus (5.7)

Triglycerides by themselves are not as powerful an indicator for the development of atherosclerosis as blood cholesterol. Alongside high LDL cholesterol levels, however, they can add considerably to the risk.

What's more, high triglycerides can enhance blood clot formation.[19] This can lead to the blockage of arteries that supply blood to the heart, brain, lungs, and limbs. They also contribute to sudden onset of angina (chest pain) in some patients.[20]

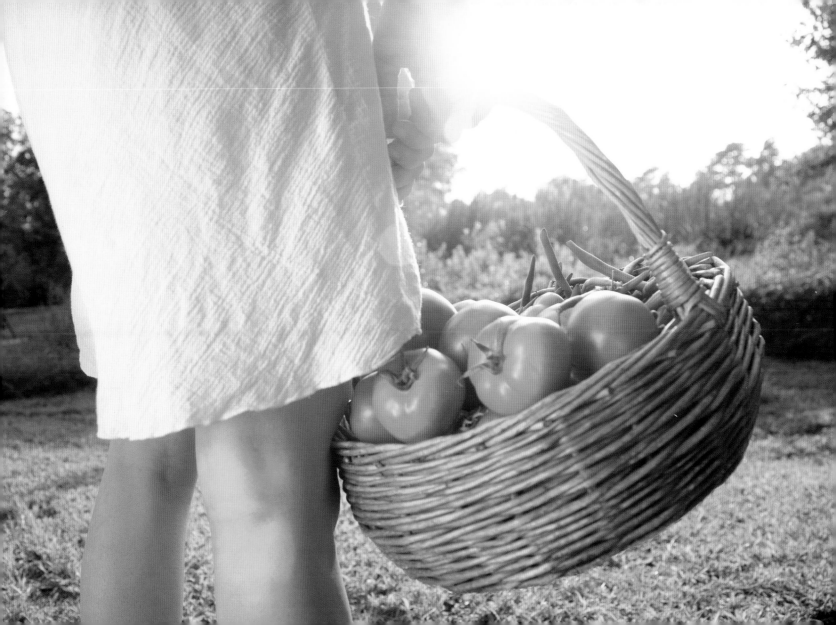

High Blood Pressure

Another significant risk factor for cardiovascular disease is high blood pressure–known medically as hypertension–contributing to half of all heart disease and strokes,[21] as well as increasing the risk of kidney disease and blindness. Worldwide, more than 1 billion people are estimated to have hypertension, with this number predicted to increase to 1.56 billion by 2025.[22] In the United States, about one in three adults have high blood pressure.[23]

Blood pressure is the force of blood against artery walls. It is measured in millimeters of mercury (mmHg) and recorded as two numbers–often expressed as systolic pressure "over" diastolic pressure. Both numbers are important indicators of risk. Blood pressure should be taken several times to get a true reading, especially for the systolic value.

Blood pressure rises and falls during the day. Your blood pressure is naturally higher when you are exerting yourself, such as during physical exercise. It is only a concern if your blood pressure is high when you are at rest, because this means your heart is overworked and your arteries have extra stress in their walls. The high force of the blood flow can also harm organs such as the heart, kidneys, brain and eyes.

In industrialized countries, rates of hypertension tend to increase with age. For example, a National Health Survey in Australia reported 14 per cent of those aged 45 to 54 years with hypertension compared with 41 per cent of those older than 75.[24]

Hypertension can be mild, moderate or severe, but most people do not know they have high blood pressure, because it usually produces no symptoms. Experts recommend that everyone should have their blood pressure checked regularly.

BLOOD PRESSURE READINGS:

Blood pressure readings are a combination of two measurements:

› **Systolic** is the highest pressure against the arteries as the heart pumps. The normal systolic pressure is between 110 and 120mmHg.

› **Diastolic** is the pressure against the arteries as the heart relaxes and fills with blood. The normal diastolic pressure is between 70 and 80mmHg.

TARGET NUMBERS (mm Hg)

	Systolic		Diastolic
Normal	less than 120	and	less than 80
Pre-hypertension	120-139	or	80-89
High	140 and above	or	90 and above

Eating up the pressure

While we don't fully understand the exact causes of high blood pressure, hereditary risk factors and stress may play a part. However, there are six definite contributing factors rooted in nutrition and lifestyle:

› Salt

Sodium chloride—commonly known as salt—is a very important contributor to hypertension. Many pre-industrialized peoples, such as Australian aborigines, tribes in Papua New Guinea and the Amazon area, people in Samoa, Africa and Central America generally consume less than 500 mg of sodium per day. And many of these societies are characterized by a total absence of hypertension. In contrast, people in industrialized nations consume between 3000 to 5000 mg of sodium per day and hypertension has a huge presence.[25]

Through a process known as osmosis, salt retains water. Excessive salt keeps the circulatory volume higher than it should be, exerting excess fluid pressure on blood vessel walls. These walls react to this stress by thickening and narrowing, leaving less space for the fluid already cramped in the blood compartment, raising "resistance" and requiring higher pressure to move blood to the organs. The heart has to pump against this high pressure system.

› Arterial plaque

As the plaques build up in our arteries, they restrict the free flow of blood. As a result, our blood pressure goes up in an effort to ensure sufficient quantities of blood circulate through ever-smaller pipelines. If the lines get too narrow and the pressure gets too high, the risks of stroke, aneurism and heart attack also increase. The principles of the optimal diet are important steps toward removing excess fat and cholesterol from our arteries, and reducing blood pressure.

Sodium chloride—commonly known as salt—is a very important contributor to hypertension.

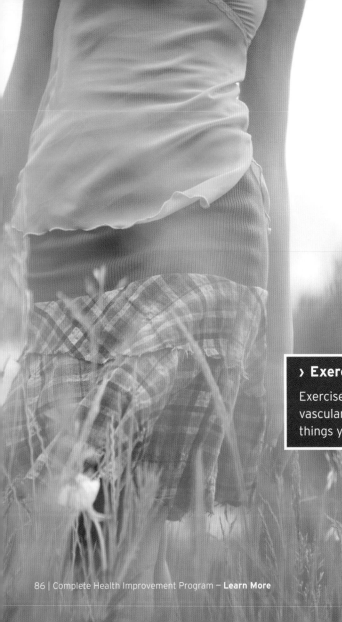

› Weight

Being overweight also directly contributes to high blood pressure. Like all the cells in our body, fat cells need to be fed and every pound of fat requires an extensive capillary system to make it functional. This means the heart requires greater pressure to get the blood through this enlarged system. Understandably, obese people are five times more likely to have hypertension.[26]

On the other hand, many people have normalized their blood pressure simply by shedding weight. Sometimes that's all it takes.

› Alcohol use

Not only is alcohol consumption linked with increased blood pressure, alcohol is also energy dense. So avoiding alcohol seems significant for bringing down blood pressure and weight levels.

› Exercise

Exercise will not only help with the daily energy balance, but it will also lower peripheral vascular resistance by making your blood flow with greater ease. One of the simplest things you can do for your overall health is go for a 30-minute walk.

› Sufficient potassium

Potassium has shown to be an important partner in battling hypertension and it helps to counteract the effects of sodium in the body.[27] Potassium is found in fresh fruits, vegetables, wholegrains and legumes. To bring down high blood pressures, we recommend nine fruits and vegetables a day.

Cutting the sodium

Many people in developed countries eat as much as 10 times the amount of salt needed. In the United States, the sodium intake for nine out of 10 adults is well above the recommended daily intake.[28]

Salt—chemically, sodium chloride—is about 40 per cent sodium, which means 1 gram of salt includes almost 400mg of sodium. It is the sodium particles in the salt that contribute to high blood pressure. In the optimal diet, sodium intake will not exceed 2000mg per day, which is equivalent to about 5 grams of salt or one teaspoon.

Sodium is a mineral found in small amounts in natural foods but only about 10 per cent of sodium intake comes from fresh food in the common modern diet. About a further 15 per cent comes from salt added to meals during cooking or at the table. The remaining 75 per cent comes from processed foods, and not necessarily from foods we would normally think of as salty. Processed meats, sauces, processed soups and stocks, breads and cereals can all contribute significant amounts of sodium.

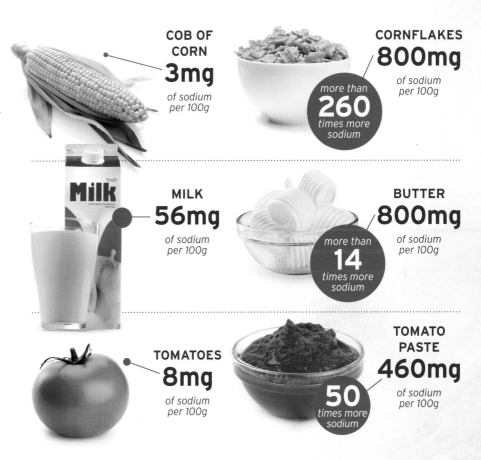

Processed foods with added sodium

COB OF CORN
3mg
of sodium per 100g

CORNFLAKES
800mg
of sodium per 100g

more than **260** times more sodium

MILK
56mg
of sodium per 100g

BUTTER
800mg
of sodium per 100g

more than **14** times more sodium

TOMATOES
8mg
of sodium per 100g

TOMATO PASTE
460mg
of sodium per 100g

50 times more sodium

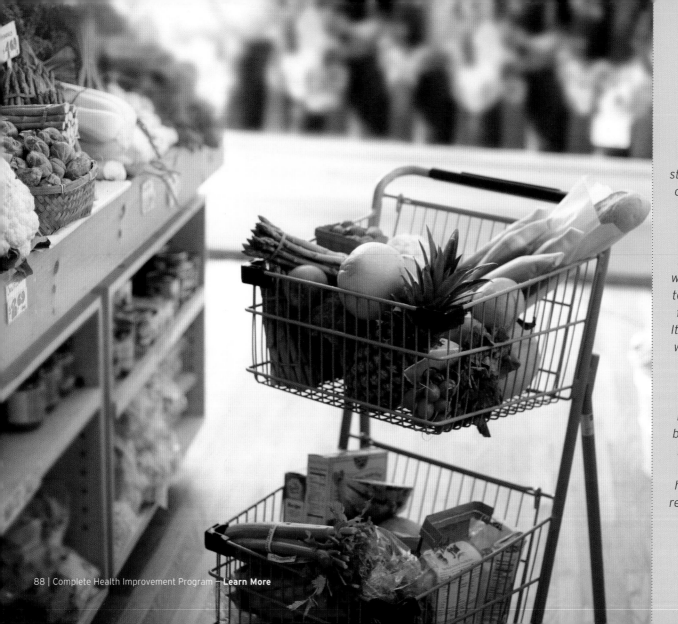

REPLACING YOUR TASTE BUDS

Taste buds are constantly being replaced on our tongues. This is good news when it comes to reducing salt in our diets because it can help with becoming accustomed to the taste of foods with less salt. It can take about four weeks to get used to a low-salt diet and, within three to six months, the palate recovers enough to be described as truly normal for the first time since infancy, helping us enjoy the real and subtle flavors of well-prepared foods.

Accordingly, reducing the amount of processed food we eat will have a significant impact on reducing our sodium intake. When we replace processed foods with fresh whole-plant foods, we are reducing a significant risk factor for high blood pressure.

Choosing low-salt products

1 Buy fresh foods and eat them without added salt.

2 Choose low salt, not "salt-reduced" foods.

3 Look at the sodium content on the nutrition information on food packaging using a standard comparative weight to compare similar products and the "per serving" column to determine how much you will actually eat.

- **Low sodium:**
  Less than 120mg/3.5oz (100g)

- **Moderate sodium:**
  Between 120-400mg/3.5oz (100g)

- **High sodium:**
  More than 400mg/3.5oz (100g)

FOOD GROUPS	SODIUM (mg)
Whole and other grains and grain products	
Cooked cereal, rice, pasta, unsalted ½ cup	0–5
Ready-to-eat cereal, 1 cup	0–360
Bread, 1 slice	110–175
Vegetables	
Fresh or frozen, cooked without salt, ½ cup	1-70
Canned or frozen with sauce, ½ cup	140–460
Tomato juice, canned, ½ cup	330
Fruit	
Fresh, frozen, canned, ½ cup	0–5
Dairy	
Milk, 1 cup	107
Yogurt, 1 cup	175
Natural cheeses, 1½ oz	110–450
Processed cheese, 2 oz	600
Nuts, seeds, and legumes	
Peanuts, salted, ⅓ cup	120
Peanuts, unsalted, ⅓ cup	0–5
Beans, cooked from dried or frozen without salt, ½ cup	0–5
Beans, canned, ½ cup	400
Lean meats, fish, and poultry	
Meat, fish, poultry, 3 oz	30–90
Tuna canned, water pack, 3 oz	230–350
Ham, lean, roasted, 3 oz	1020

The optimal lifestyle for heart health

Despite the prevalence of heart disease in developed nations and increasingly the rest of the world, the optimal lifestyle offers hope for reducing the greatest risks for the development of cardiovascular disease. By recommending a low-fat, high-fiber eating pattern focused on unprocessed whole plant foods, the optimal diet reduces risks associated with cholesterol and high blood pressure in a number of important ways. When combined with regular physical activity, other risks such as unhealthy body weight are also significantly reduced. In contrast with medication, the optimal lifestyle is a prescription with no potential risk of side effects or complications.

KEY POINTS

› Cardiovascular disease is the leading cause of death in the world today.

› High cholesterol and high blood pressure are significant risk factors to heart health.

› The optimal diet—including a wide range of whole plant-based foods—reduces and counteracts many of the dietary hazards that contribute to raised cholesterol and blood pressure.

Chapter Six References

1. Lamon, B D, and D P Hajjar (2008), "Inflammation at the Molecular Interface of Atherogenesis," *American Journal of Pathology,* Vol 173 No 5, pages 1253-64.

2. World Health Organization (2011), "The top 10 causes of death. Fact sheet number 310.".

3. Napoli, C, et al (2006), "Nitric oxide and atherosclerosis: an update," *Nitric Oxide,* Vol 15 No 4, pages 265-79.

4. National Heart Lung and Blood Institute (2011), "What is Atherosclerosis?" <http://www.nhlbi.nih.gov/health/health-topics/topics/atherosclerosis/>.

5. McGill, H C, et al (2000), "Origin of atherosclerosis in childhood and adolescence," *American Journal of Clinical Nutrition,* Vol 72 No 5 Supplement, pages 1307S-15S.

6. National Heart Lung and Blood Institute (2011), "What is Cholesterol?" <http://www.nhlbi.nih.gov/health/health-topics/topics/hbc/>.

7. Better Health Channel (2012), "Cholesterol," <http://www.betterhealth.vic.gov.au/bhcv2/bhcarticles.nsf/pages/cholesterol_explained>.

8. Stamler, J, et al (1986), "Is relationship between serum cholesterol and risk of premature death from coronary heart disease continuous and graded? Findings in 356,222 primary screenees of the Multiple Risk Factor Intervention Trial (MRFIT)," *Journal of the American Medical Association,* Vol 256 No 20, pages 2823-8.

9. National Cholesterol Education Program (NCEP) Expert Panel (2002), "Third Report of the National Cholesterol Education Program (NCEP) Expert Panel on Detection, Evaluation, and Treatment of High Blood Cholesterol in

Adults (Adult Treatment Panel III) final report," *Circulation*, Vol 106 No 25, pages 3143–421.

10 Lamon and Hajjar (2008), op cit.

11 Manson, J E, et al (1992), "The Primary Prevention of Myocardial Infarction," *New England Journal of Medicine*, Vol 326 No 21, pages 1406–14.

12 Englert, H S, H A Diehl and R L Greenlaw (2004), "Rationale and design of the Rockford CHIP, a community-based coronary risk reduction program: results of a pilot phase," Preventive Medicine, Vol 38, pages 432–41; Rankin P, D P Morton, H A Diehl, et al (2012), "Effectiveness of a Volunteer-Delivered Lifestyle Modification Program for Reducing Cardiovascular Disease Risk Factors," *American Journal of Cardiology*, Vol 109, No 1, pages 82–6.

13 Judd, J T, et al (1994), "Dietary trans fatty acids: effects on plasma lipids and lipoproteins of healthy men and women," *American Journal of Clinical Nutrition*, Vol 59 No 4, pages 861–8.

14 Heart Foundation (2009), "Saturated and trans fats," <http://www.heartfoundation.org.au/SiteCollectionDocuments/Dietary-Fats-Dietary-Cholesterol-and-Heart-Health.pdf>.

15 West, S G (2001), "Effect of diet on vascular reactivity: an emerging marker for vascular risk," *Current Atherosclerosis Reports*, Vol 3 No 6, pages 446–55.

16 Ripsin, C M, et al (1992), "Oat products and lipid lowering. A meta-analysis," *Journal of the American Medical Association*, Vol 267 No 24, pages 3317–25.

17 Couillard, C, et al (2001), "Effects of Endurance Exercise Training on Plasma HDL Cholesterol Levels Depend on Levels of Triglycerides: Evidence From Men of the Health, Risk Factors, Exercise Training and Genetics (HERITAGE) Family Study," *Arteriosclerosis, Thrombosis, and Vascular Biology*, Vol 21 No 7, pages 1226–32.

18 Kasapis, C, and P D Thompson (2005), "The effects of physical activity on serum C-reactive protein and inflammatory markers: a systematic review," *Journal of the American College of Cardiology*, Vol 45 No 10, pages 1563–9.

19 Varbo, A, et al (2011), "Nonfasting triglycerides, cholesterol and ischemic stroke in the general population," *Annals of Neurology*, Vol 69 No 4, pages 628–34.

20 Borge, G, et al (2007), "Nonfasting Triglycerides and Risk of Myocardial Infarction, Ischemic Heart Disease and Death in Men and Women," *Journal of the American Medical Association*, Vol 298 No 3, pages 299–308.

21 Australian Division of World Action on Salt and Health (2011), "How Much Salt are we Eating?" <www.awash.org.au>.

22 Kearney, P M, et al (2005), "Global burden of hypertension: analysis of worldwide data," *Lancet*, Vol 365 No 9455, page 217–23.

23 Centers for Disease Control and Prevention (2011), "Vital signs: prevalence, treatment, and control of hypertension—United States, 1999-2002 and 2005-2008," *Morbidity and Mortality Weekly Report*, Vol 60 No 4, pages 103–8.

24 Australian Bureau of Statistics (2006), "Cardiovascular Disease in Australia: A Snapshot, 2004–05," <www.abs.gov.au/ausstats/abs@.nsf/mf/4821.0.55.001>.

25 Brown, I J, et al (2009), "Salt intakes around the world: implications for public health," *International Journal of Epidemiology*, Vol 38 No 3, pages 791–813.

26 Haslam, D W, and W P James (2005), "Obesity," *Lancet*, Vol 366 No 9492, pages 1197–209.

27 The INTERSALT Co-operative Research Group (1988), "Sodium, potassium, body mass, alcohol and blood pressure: the INTERSALT Study," *Journal of Hypertension Supplement*, Vol 6 No 4, pages S584–6.

28 Centre for Disease Control and Prevention (2010), "Sodium Intake Among Adults—United States, 2005-2006," *Journal of the American Medical Association*, Vol 304 No 7, pages 738–40.

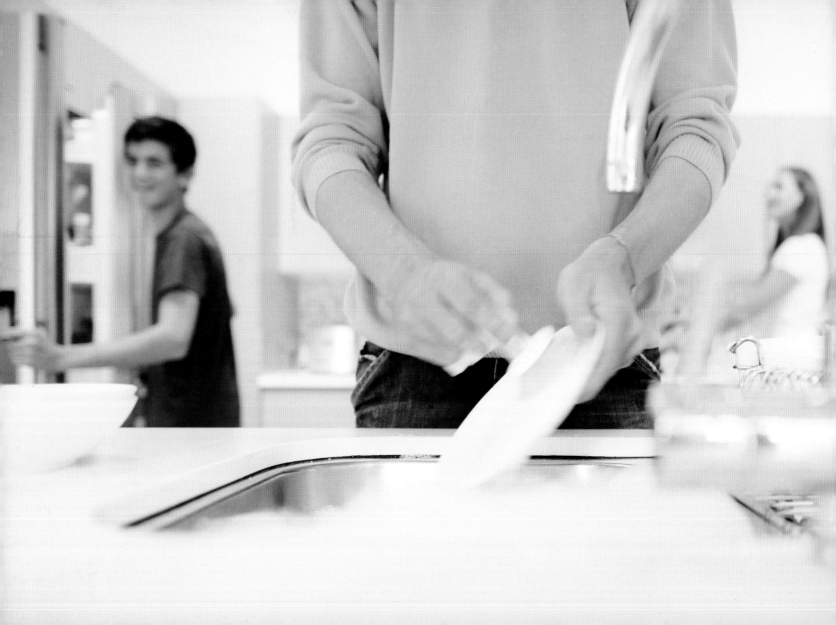

Chapter Seven

Disarming Diabetes

Don't you just hate it when something that worked fine for years suddenly stops working? Like that kitchen drain that clogs up. Only when the sink won't empty anymore do you realize how much you took functional plumbing for granted. It's harder to prepare food without the sink, maybe the kitchen starts to smell, and every time you turn around to wash your hands you realize you now have to walk upstairs.

You didn't realize one blocked drain could annoy you in so many ways.

You have to work hard to get the drain flowing again, plunger in hand, you're covered in gunk you don't even want to know the origin of. Maybe you even have to call in a professional to fix it for you if the problem is too serious.

After it's working again, you might sit back and realize it was something you were putting down the drain that clogged it. Perhaps the plumber tells you it was something you didn't even know you shouldn't put down the drain. Either way, you're going to be more careful about it from now on. You know how hard it was to fix the problem—much more difficult than just stopping it from happening.

In many ways, lifestyle diseases such as diabetes are like that drain. We often take our health for granted until it starts being affected. Only then we realize the enormous impact small side effects can have on our day-to-day lives.

While the problem seems to appear all of a sudden, it has been building for some time and we realize we have been, usually unknowingly, slowly contributing to this all along.

But, like that clogged drain, the good news is there are things we can do to stop lifestyle diseases from taking hold—and things we can do to get our bodies working again!

We often take our health for granted until it starts being affected.

What is diabetes?

In simple terms, diabetes is when the body is no longer able to produce insulin or when the insulin produced is no longer effective in moving glucose from the blood stream into cells, where it is needed. There are different types of diabetes, but when we talk about diabetes caused by lifestyle choices, we are referring to type 2 diabetes. Higher risk of type 2 diabetes is associated with being overweight, being inactive, and consuming diets high in red meat and low in fiber.

Common symptoms of diabetes include:[1]

- Excessive thirst
- Frequent urination
- Extreme hunger
- Unusual weight loss
- Increased fatigue
- Irritability
- Blurred vision
- Slow-healing wounds
- Recurring infections

Complications due to poorly controlled diabetes can be very serious, including blindness and limb amputation.[2] Diabetes is a major risk factor for kidney disease and impotence. It also greatly increases the risk of cardiovascular disease and stroke, as elevated blood sugar levels cause damage to the large and small blood vessels of the body.[3] It is estimated that a diagnosis of diabetes represents a reduction in life expectancy of 12 to 14 years.[4]

And not all people with diabetes may know they have it. For instance, of the 25.8 million people affected by diabetes in the United States population, only 18.8 million have been diagnosed,[5] meaning there are many people who are suffering the increased health risks that come with diabetes without being aware of it or having an opportunity to improve their health.

DIABETES: WHICH TYPE?

90%
TYPE 2 DIABETES

5%
TYPE 1 DIABETES

5%
GESTATIONAL DIABETES

TYPE 1 DIABETES

Referred to in the past as juvenile-onset diabetes or insulin-dependent diabetes, affects about 5 per cent of diabetes cases. While the exact cause of type 1 diabetes is not known, it is thought that an environmental factor, such as a virus, may cause the immune system to attack insulin-producing cells in the pancreas. Sufferers are left without the ability to produce insulin, resulting in an inability for glucose to find its way out of the blood and into cells. Those with type 1 diabetes must regularly take injections of insulin to replace that which the body can no longer make. While lifestyle choices such as poor diet or lack of physical activity are not the cause of type 1 diabetes, they can have a significant impact on the management of symptoms.[7]

GESTATIONAL DIABETES

A temporary form of diabetes that develops in some women during pregnancy, which accounts for about 5 per cent of diagnosed cases of diabetes. Those who suffer from gestational diabetes are at an increased risk of developing type 2 diabetes later in life. However, the good news is positive lifestyle behaviors can reduce this risk.

TYPE 2 DIABETES

This type of diabetes is 90 per cent of diabetes cases and will be the focus of this chapter. It is a lifestyle disease, strongly associated with other health conditions, such as heart disease, obesity, high blood cholesterol and high blood pressure. Type 2 diabetes occurs when the body's cells no longer effectively respond to insulin and the pancreas cannot produce enough insulin to meet this increased need. Type 2 diabetes can be prevented and studies have also shown some symptoms may be reversed and blood sugar levels normalized using healthy eating and physical activity.[8] In the past, type 2 diabetes has been referred to as adult-onset diabetes or non-insulin-dependent diabetes. However, over the past two decades, type 2 diabetes has started presenting in children and severe cases calling for insulin therapy are not uncommon, rendering both labels unsuitable.

Diagnosing type 2 diabetes by the numbers

Pre-diabetes and type 2 diabetes are considered progressive variations of the same dysfunction. While the best medicine is prevention, implementing dietary and lifestyle factors at any stage can help halt the progression, and reverse symptoms and underlying causes. In the United States, the following criteria are used in the identification of these conditions:

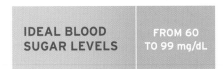

IDEAL BLOOD SUGAR LEVELS	FROM 60 TO 99 mg/dL

▲ Fasting plasma glucose from 60 to 99 mg/dL (3.3-5.5mmol/L).

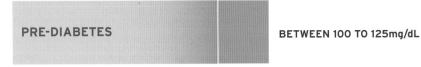

PRE-DIABETES	BETWEEN 100 TO 125mg/dL

▲ Fasting plasma glucose of between 100 to 125mg/dL (5.6-6.9mmol/L)

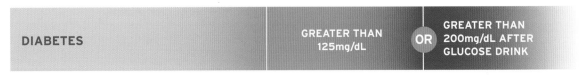

DIABETES	GREATER THAN 125mg/dL	OR	GREATER THAN 200mg/dL AFTER GLUCOSE DRINK

▲ Two consecutive tests with fasting plasma glucose concentrations greater than or equal to 125mg/dL (7mmol/L) or greater than or equal to 200mg/dL (11.1mmol/L) 2 hours after a 2.65oz (75g) glucose drink

While the best medicine is prevention, implementing dietary and lifestyle factors at any stage can help halt the progression and reverse symptoms.

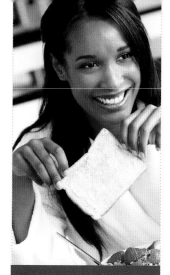

TRY THIS:

Enzymes in saliva start breaking down carbohydrate in our mouths as soon as we start chewing a food. Try chewing a piece of regular bread. If you chew long enough, the savory complex carbohydrates will slowly turn sweeter in your mouth as the enzymes go to work!

How does sugar get into the blood?

Among the thousands of compounds they contain, foods and drinks can provide us with macro nutrients that our body can use for energy. One of these macro nutrients is carbohydrate, the preferred fuel source for our bodies.

Carbohydrates are found in foods in a variety of forms, but the building blocks for all carbohydrates are simple molecules we often refer to as sugars. Foods high in carbohydrates include bread, legumes, cereals and grains, pasta, starchy vegetables, fruits and high-sugar products, such as fruits juices, sodas or soft drinks.

When we eat a carbohydrate-rich food—whether it has long, complex carbohydrate molecules or simple sugars—the body must break these down into their simplest form before they can be absorbed by the small intestine and find their way into our blood. Our blood is used as the transport system to get this sugar (glucose) to the far reaches of our body, so it can be delivered to the cells of our muscles and organs to power them throughout the day. While all carbohydrates are broken down into the same simple molecules, other components of food will influence how quickly this happens. Fiber—a crucial component of unprocessed plant foods—also plays a key role in this process, helping moderate the rate at which carbohydrates are absorbed, making unprocessed plant foods the best carbohydrate foods available.

Preventing diabetes

When it comes to preventing diabetes, our first line of defense is lifestyle—what we put in our mouths and how much we move. These two components are incredibly powerful and research has shown that these can be more effective in preventing type 2 diabetes than the most commonly prescribed diabetes medication.[10] When you think about it, this makes sense: if lifestyle contributes to this disease, then the answer to fighting it can also be found in our lifestyle.

While the advice "move more" is self explanatory, things seem more complicated as we move into the area of food. Over the years, there have been many differing recommendations for the "diabetic diet" involving complicated assessments of foods and calculations before meals. But the good news is that research points us toward a simpler approach to diet that achieves fantastic results. It points toward an eating pattern that's not a "diabetic diet" but an optimal way of eating for everyone.

› Diet

You might be thinking that the only thing in the diet we need to look out for is going to be sugar. After all, we want to control sugar levels in the blood, so it seems cutting sugar out of the diet should fix this.

Refined carbohydrates are certainly not our friend when it comes to diabetes, but research indicates they are not the only thing we need to be looking out for. While we want to control sugar levels in the blood, another component of food may interfere with how our body deals with carbohydrates. If we can address this and choose good sources of carbohydrates, our body is better able to deal with the carbohydrates we are receiving from food.

Like many things in nutritional science, there is some uncertainty as to exactly how fat interferes with how our body uses glucose. There are a number of theories around this and new research brings us closer to answering this question. But what is clear from decades of research is that low-fat diets, high in fiber and unrefined carbohydrates, cannot just reduce the risk of developing diabetes, but may also cause a reversal of some symptoms and normalisation of blood sugar levels in those diagnosed with the disease.

When choosing a good carbohydrate-rich food, look for those that are minimally processed.

› The facts on fat

A number of research studies have demonstrated the dramatic difference a low-fat, high-fiber diet can make in the health of people already diagnosed with diabetes.

Australian researcher Dr Karen O'Dea took a group of 10 Aboriginal people back to their traditional lifestyle and diet. They were all urbanized and diagnosed diabetics but, over a period of seven weeks, they lived as hunter-gatherers in the Australian outback.

With a diet consisting largely of roots, berries and wild animals, the fat content was 13 per cent of the average 1200 calories (5000 kilojoules) they consumed each day. In the process, they lost an average of 18 pounds (8 kilograms) and their average diabetic blood sugars of 209 mg/dL (11.6 mmol/L) dropped to non-diabetic levels of 119 mg/dL (6.6 mmol/L) without having to rely on any medication. The difference was a simple, less refined, more traditional diet with little fat and lots of fiber.[11]

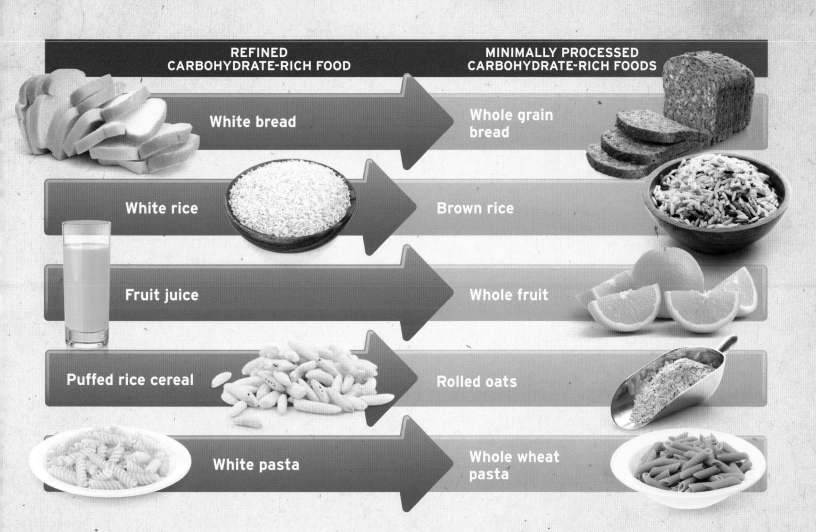

REFINED CARBOHYDRATE-RICH FOOD → **MINIMALLY PROCESSED CARBOHYDRATE-RICH FOODS**

White bread → Whole grain bread

White rice → Brown rice

Fruit juice → Whole fruit

Puffed rice cereal → Rolled oats

White pasta → Whole wheat pasta

A more recent study with similar results was that conducted by Dr Neal Barnard. Type 2 diabetes patients were put on either a low-fat, plant-based diet or a diet recommended by the American Diabetes Association. Both groups of patients saw improvements in their glycemic control but those on the lower-fat diet saw greater results. The plant-based diet had no cholesterol, it was very low in fat, and there were almost no saturated fats or trans fats. The diet was also high in fiber, high in antioxidants, low in calorie density and the patients were not restricted in the amount of food they could choose to eat, they just limited their choices to minimally processed foods. Of these patients, 71 per cent no longer required medication after 30 days.[12]

› Questioning carbohydrates

While carbohydrate-rich foods are not the cause of diabetes, there are still good and bad choices when it comes to carbohydrate-rich foods, and identifying them is simple. When choosing a good carbohydrate-rich food, look for those that are minimally processed. These foods generally come with all their fiber, vitamins and minerals, as compared to their refined cousins.

A good example of this is corn—a whole plant food that's naturally full of fiber, vitamins and minerals. By comparison, cornstarch is a highly processed corn product that has almost all its fiber removed, along with large amounts of other nutrients.

Many food companies who produce processed foods try to add back or "fortify" their foods with some of the vitamins and minerals removed during processing. But given the complex nature of food, we probably cannot even identify all the things we remove from a food during processing, so we can't add them all back in. We would do better simply to leave them in.

› Whole grains

Higher intakes of cereal fiber and whole grains typical of a vegetarian diet have been associated with a reduced risk of type 2 diabetes in several studies. These grains have nutrients that protect against the development of diabetes and work to reduce the risks of diabetes in those already diagnosed.[13] However, the health benefits of these whole grains are further enhanced by the fact that they often replace more harmful foods in the diet.

Care should be taken when purchasing premade grain foods, such as bread. A label describing a product as whole wheat, wholemeal, wholegrain or multigrain does not guarantee the nutritional value of the product. Check the ingredients labels for information about what percentages of the products are what they claim to be.

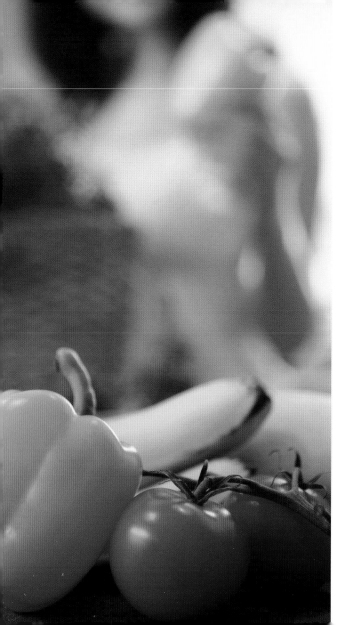

› Red meat

Three studies of diet and diabetes based at Harvard University tracked the dietary habits of 200,000 people over the period of a decade and found a strong association between consumption of red meat and increased risk of type 2 diabetes.

The studies found that 4 oz (100g) of unprocessed red meat per day increased diabetes risk by 20 per cent. Similarly, 2 oz (50g) of processed red meat per day—including products such as bacon, hot dogs and sausages—increased the diabetes risk by 50 per cent. By contrast, when one serving of processed red meat per day was replaced with a wholegrain dish, the diabetes risk dropped by as much as 35 per cent.[14]

Again, the researchers were unclear as to exactly why meat should have such a strong impact on the risk of developing type 2 diabetes but suggested three possible explanations:

- Weight gain.
- Toxic effect of nitrosamines on the insulin-producing pancreatic cells.
- The oxidative stress and inflammation related to the kind of iron in meat and the way it is prepared.

DIABETES MEDICATIONS

While the first advice for treating or preventing type 2 diabetes is diet and lifestyle, if the disease progresses, often a range of medications are used to help manage blood sugar levels within an acceptable range.

A recent report found that of the diagnosed diabetics 58 per cent are on pills, 12 per cent are on insulin injections, 14 per cent are using both, and 16 per cent are on some kind of diabetic diet.[15]

While insulin and medications can control the blood sugar, insulin and many medications also tend to stimulate the appetite, risking further weight gain, in turn increasing the need for more insulin and medication.

While these medications can be helpful in limiting the damage that can be caused by continuously high blood sugar levels, they do not represent a cure and come with their own range of potential side effects. As with all medications, it is important to work in partnership with your physician regarding the use of diabetes medications to ensure optimal health outcomes. Medications should never be discontinued without consultation with your physician.

Beating diabetes

As the rates of diabetes continue to grow alarmingly around the world, the answer is simple. With good lifestyle choices—particularly healthy diet and regular activity—the risks of developing type 2 diabetes can be dramatically reduced. We do not need to wait for the drain to be clogged to begin clearing it out.

Armed with those same lifestyle choices and with the supervision of their doctor or physician, most diabetes patients should be able to reduce their dependence on medication and potentially reverse this chronic and dangerous disease.

It's a matter of choice—and the many smaller choices we make each day.

KEY POINTS

› Type 2 diabetes accounts for 90 per cent of diabetes cases and development of this chronic disease is growing to epidemic levels around the world.

› Diabetes is the body's inability to properly process and deliver sugars in the blood stream, which in turn causes other damage to the body.

› Diets high in fat, which also include unnecessary sugar and the consumption of red meat, contribute significantly to the risks of developing diabetes.

Chapter Seven References

1   Clark, N G, K M Fox, and S Grandy (2007), "Symptoms of diabetes and their association with the risk and presence of diabetes: findings from the Study to Help Improve Early evaluation and management of risk factors Leading to Diabetes (SHIELD)," *Diabetes Care,* Vol 30 No 11, pages 2868-73.

2   Hiatt, W R, et al (1990), "Diagnostic methods for peripheral arterial disease in the San Luis Valley Diabetes Study," Journal of Clinical Epidemiology, Vol 43 No 6, pages 597-606; Reiber, G E, R E Pecoraro, and T D Koepsell (1992), "Risk factors for amputation in patients with diabetes mellitus. A case-control study," Annals of Internal Medicine, Vol 117 No 2, pages 97-105; Tapp, R J, et al (2003), "The prevalence of and factors associated with diabetic retinopathy in the Australian population," *Diabetes Care,* Vol 26 No 6, pages 1731-7.

3   Kannel, W B, and D L McGee (1979), "Diabetes and cardiovascular disease. The Framingham study," Journal of the American Medical Association, Vol 241 No 19, pages 2035-8; Yusuf, S, et al (2004), "Effect of potentially modifiable risk factors associated with myocardial infarction in 52 countries (the INTERHEART study): case-control study," *Lancet,* Vol 364 No 9438, pages 937-52.

4. Narayan, K M, et al (2003), "Lifetime risk for diabetes mellitus in the United States," *Journal of the American Medical Association,* Vol 290 No 14, pages 1884-90.

5   National diabetes Fact Sheet, 2011, <www.cdc.gov/diabetes>, accessed August, 2011.

6   Ahmed, A M (2002), "History of diabetes mellitus," *Saudi Medical Journal,* Vol 23 No 4, pages 373-8."

7   Wasserman, D H, and B Zinman (1994), "Exercise in individuals with IDDM," *Diabetes Care,* Vol 17 No 8, pages 924-37.

8   Hu, F B, et al (2001), "Diet, lifestyle, and the risk of type 2 diabetes mellitus in women," *New England Journal of Medicine,* Vol 345 No 11, pages 790-7; Barnard, N D, et al (2006), "A low-fat vegan diet improves glycemic control and cardiovascular risk factors in a randomized clinical trial in individuals with type 2 diabetes," *Diabetes Care,* Vol 29 No 8, pages 1777-83.

9   World Health Organization (2006), "Definition and diagnosis of diabetes mellitus and intermediate hyperglycemia," WHO/IDF consultation.

10 Knowler, W C, et al (2002), "Reduction in the incidence of type 2 diabetes with lifestyle intervention or metformin," *New England Journal of Medicine,* Vol 346 No 6, pages 393-403.

11 O'Dea, K (1984), "Marked improvement in carbohydrate and lipid metabolism in diabetic Australian aborigines after temporary reversion to traditional lifestyle," *Diabetes,* Vol 33 No 6, pages 596-603.

12 Barnard, N D, et al (2006), "A low-fat vegan diet improves glycemic control and cardiovascular risk factors in a randomized clinical trial in individuals with type 2 diabetes," *Diabetes Care,* Vol 29 No 8, page 1777-83.

13 Marsh, K, and J Brand-Miller (2011), "Vegetarian Diets and Diabetes," *American Journal of Lifestyle Medicine,* Vol 5, pages 135-43.

14 Pan, A, et al (2011), "Red meat consumption and risk of type 2 diabetes: 3 cohorts of US adults and an updated meta-analysis," *American Journal of Clinical Nutrition,* Vol 94 No 4, pages 1088-96.

15 Diseases, N.I.o.D.a.D.a.K. "National Diabetes Statistics, 2011," <http://diabetes.niddk.nih.gov/dm/pubs/statistics>.

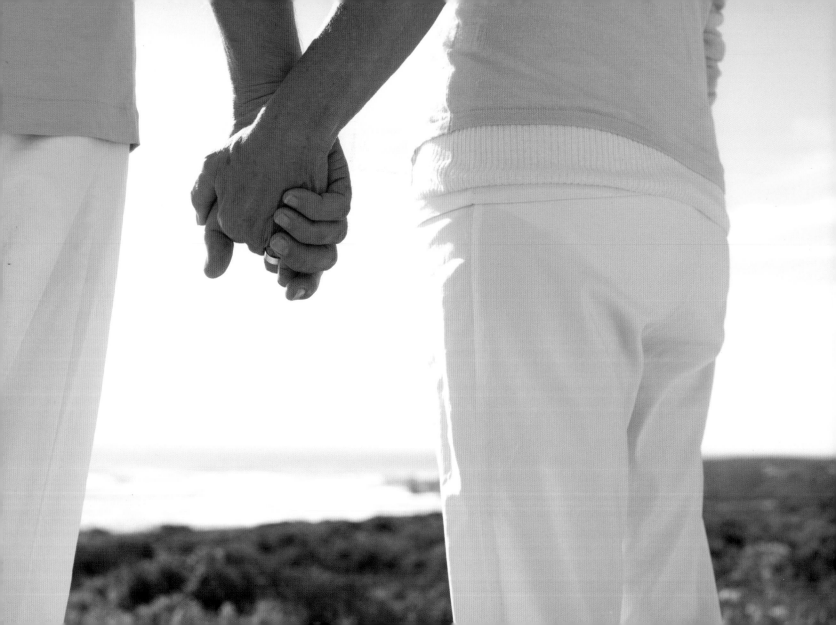

Chapter Eight

Cancer Prevention

Cancer is a frightening subject. In many developed countries, it is difficult to find someone who hasn't had a friend or loved one whose life has been touched by this devastating disease. While research continues to search for the best ways to combat this disease, you may be surprised to know that science has done some impressive work identifying factors that can contribute to our risk of cancer. It might not be a surprise to you that many of them are lifestyle related.

The World Cancer Research Fund (WCRF) is a not-for-profit association that leads and unifies a global network of charities dedicated to funding research and education programs into the link between food, nutrition, weight maintenance and cancer risk.

Their second "Expert Report" was published in 2007 and is possibly the most comprehensive book ever published on the links between food, nutrition, physical activity and cancer prevention, and is based on in-depth analysis of more than 7000 scientific studies published on cancer prevention during the past 50 years.[1]

As part of this report, the WCRF developed eight personal recommendations, which the authors believe can decrease an individual's risk of developing a number of different types of cancer.

Following are those eight recommendations, with explanations of how they can fit within the optimal lifestyle.

Science has done some impressive work identifying factors that can contribute to our risk of cancer.

WHAT IS CANCER?

Our cells are growing and renewing themselves every day, with this process being controlled by the cells' genetic blueprint. If something causes a mistake to occur in this genetic blueprint, this cell growth can get out of control. Cancer is the name used to describe groups of these out-of-control cells growing and possibly spreading inside the body. Cancerous cells can originate from any type of tissue in the body, which means many different types of cancer can occur.

Cancer cells that do not spread beyond the immediate area in which they start growing are said to be benign, which means they are not considered dangerous. If cancer cells spread into surrounding areas or different parts of the body, they are called malignant and commonly referred to as cancer.

A mass of these abnormal cells is called a tumor. Cancer cells can break away from a tumor and travel around the body via the bloodstream or lymphatic system to different parts of the body. If these cells settle in other parts of the body, they can form a secondary cancer or metastasis. Cancer can be deadly because it can stop parts of the body, such as vital organs, from working properly.

While some substances have been identified as cancer-causing—referred to as carcinogens—we do not know all the possible risks and causes for cancer. However, research has identified a range of lifestyle behaviors that can raise or lower the risk of a range of different types of cancer.

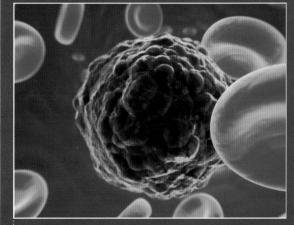

› Cancer is the name used to describe groups of out-of-control cells growing and possibly spreading inside the body.

According to the World Health Organization, cancer accounted for 7.6 million deaths world-wide in 2008, with this figure expected to rise to 13.1 million by 2030. Lung, stomach, liver, colon and breast cancer cause the most cancer deaths each year, with about 30 per cent of cancer deaths being due to five leading behavioral and dietary risk factors: overweight or obese, low fruit and vegetable intake, lack of physical activity, tobacco use and alcohol use.[2]

Recommendation 1: Body fatness

> Be as lean as possible within the normal range of body weight.

Personal Recommendations

> Ensure that body weight through childhood and adolescent growth projects toward the lower end of the normal Body Mass Index range at age 21.

> Maintain body weight within the normal range from age 21.

> Avoid weight gain and increases in waist circumference throughout adulthood.

The WCRF found that maintaining a healthy weight throughout life may be one of the most important ways to protect against cancer—which is all about a healthy lifestyle. On-and-off dieting leads to on-and-off weight gain. A diet based on whole plant foods is less energy dense than a modern diet full of fats and sugar, making it harder to over-consume energy and easier to maintain a healthy body weight.

One specific type of cancer associated with body fatness is breast cancer. In China, the association between being overweight at the time of or soon after breast cancer diagnosis and survival was investigated in 1455 patients aged 25 to 64 from the Shanghai Breast Cancer Study. The investigators found that being overweight at diagnosis or soon afterward was associated with poorer overall survival and disease-free survival. This finding held up, even when the researchers adjusted for age and other risk factors for breast cancer. This suggests that body fatness may be an independent risk factor for breast cancer.[3]

Being overweight at cancer diagnosis or soon afterward was associated with poorer overall survival and disease-free survival.

Recommendation 2:
Physical activity

> Be physically active as part of everyday life.

Personal Recommendations

> Be moderately physically active, equivalent to brisk walking, for at least 30 minutes every day.

> As fitness improves, aim for 60 minutes or more of moderate physical activity or for 30 minutes or more of vigorous physical activity every day.

> Limit sedentary habits such as watching television.

The WCRF found that most populations and people living in industrialized and urban settings have habitually low activity levels. The optimal lifestyle promotes a range of different types of physical activity for optimal health and wellbeing. Cancer prevention is just another great reason to get active!

Cancer prevention is just another great reason to get active!

There is evidence to suggest that physical activity, when combined with healthy eating, may be a powerful protector from cancer. One great example is a study from California, which studied 1490 women diagnosed and treated for early-stage breast cancer. The investigators were looking at these women to try to find any associations that might exist between physical activity, diet and obesity, and survival after breast cancer.

The researchers found that those women consuming five or more daily servings of vegetables and fruits, and doing physical activity equivalent to 30 minutes of walking six days a week had a significant survival advantage. Perhaps surprisingly, the researchers also found that these women gained this survival advantage regardless of whether they were a healthy weight or obese. This research suggests that, regardless of weight, there may be amazing benefits to be gained from adopting a healthy lifestyle.[4]

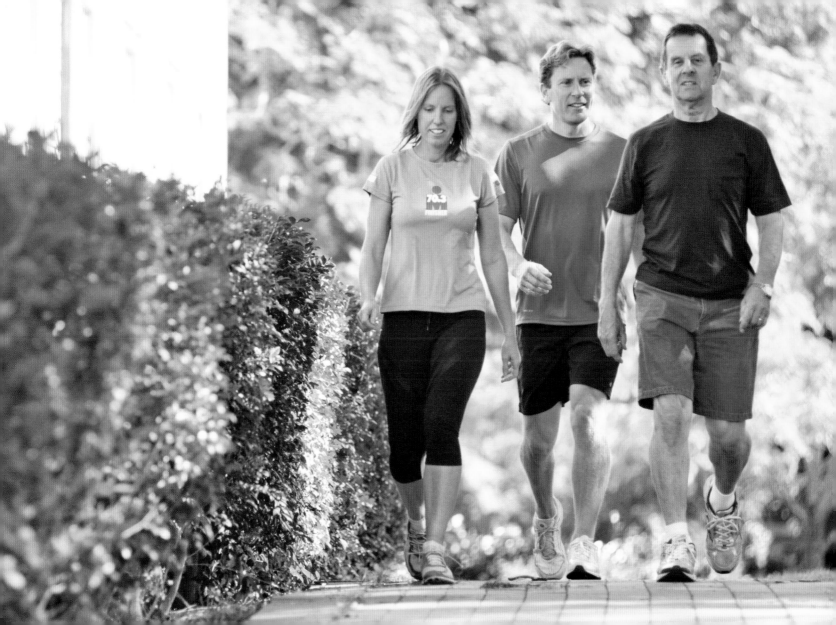

Juicy goodness?

Sugar content per 8-ounce (250ml) serving, all juices are unsweetened

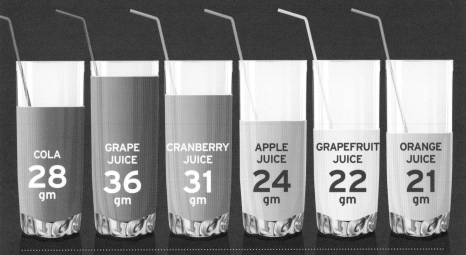

COLA	GRAPE JUICE	CRANBERRY JUICE	APPLE JUICE	GRAPEFRUIT JUICE	ORANGE JUICE
28 gm	36 gm	31 gm	24 gm	22 gm	21 gm

You may know that a standard 8-oz (250ml) glass of cola can contain as much as 7 teaspoons (about 28 grams) of sugar, but did you know some fruit juices can contain this much as well?[5] Many people think fruit juice is a great beverage choice, but they can contain as many calories as some fizzy drinks. While it is true they contain some vitamins and minerals and their sugar is naturally occurring, rather than added, this is the same for the whole fruit, which is more difficult to overeat due to its high dietary fiber content, much of which is removed in the juicing process. So remember, water should always be your first-choice drink as part of an optimal lifestyle.

Recommendation 3: Foods and drinks that promote weight gain

> Limit consumption of energy-dense foods.

> Avoid sugary drinks.

Personal Recommendations

> Consume energy-dense foods sparingly.

> Avoid sugary drinks.

> Consume "fast foods" sparingly, if at all.

The WCRF found that consumption of energy-dense foods and sugary drinks is increasing worldwide and is probably contributing to the global increase in obesity. The optimal diet is all about filling up on nutrient-dense, energy-sparse foods, with water as the beverage of choice.

Recommendation 4: Plant foods

› Eat mostly foods of plant origin.

Personal Recommendations

› Eat at least five portions/servings (at least 14 oz or 400g) of a variety of vegetables and fruits every day.

› Eat relatively unprocessed cereals (grains) and/or pulses (legumes) with every meal.

› Limit refined starchy foods.

› People who consume starchy roots or tubers as staples should also ensure intake of sufficient vegetables, fruits and pulses (legumes).

The WCRF found that the evidence shows that most diets that are protective against cancer are made up mostly of plant origin. The optimal diet is all about whole plant foods. These amazing foods, when eaten as grown, provide a fantastic range of nutrients to help keep our bodies nourished and in top condition. The WCRF specifically points toward diets that give an emphasis to plant foods that are high in nutrients, high in dietary fiber and low in energy density.

THE GOODNESS OF SOY

A number of research studies have linked soy consumption with a lower risk of breast cancer. A review of studies, published in the British Journal of Cancer in 2008 found that among high soy-consuming Asian women, there appeared to be a significant trend of decreasing breast cancer risk with increasing soy food intake. Soy consumption was categorized by the level of soy isoflavones participants ate on an average day, with those in the highest group consuming a similar amount of isoflavones to what could be found in 30 fl oz (900ml) of soy milk. In contrast, soy intake appeared to be unrelated to breast cancer risk in studies looking at low soy-consuming Western populations, whose highest average intake levels of isoflavones were equivalent to about 1 fl oz (30ml) of soy milk daily. The authors concluded that soy intake in the amount consumed in Asian populations may have protective effects against breast cancer.[6] While research in the area of soy consumption and breast cancer is ongoing, this research suggests that Western populations may be able to receive potential benefits from increasing consumption of soy to levels comparable to those consumed by high soy-consuming Asian women.

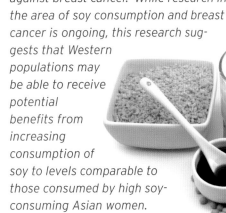

The healthy eating continuum emphasizes that better health outcomes come with reducing meat consumption.

Recommendation 5: Animal foods

› Limit intake of red meat and avoid processed meat.

Personal Recommendation

› People who eat red meat should consume less than 18 oz (500g) per week, with very little—if any—to be processed meats.

The WCRF states that "red or processed meats are convincing or probable causes of some cancers" and that "diets with high levels of animal fats are often relatively high in energy, increasing the risk of weight gain."

The healthy eating continuum emphasizes that better health outcomes come with reducing meat consumption, with the far end of the continuum being eliminating it from the diet completely. However, the WCRF's focus on a range of lifestyle factors is another reason we promote the optimal lifestyle, aiming for improvement across all areas of lifestyle to see the greatest benefits.

Cancer research is an ever-evolving area of study, with exciting new research coming out every day, expanding our knowledge of this disease and its prevention. One particular area that has shown early promising results through the use of lifestyle medicine is prostate cancer. Dr Dean Ornish, a pioneer of lifestyle medicine, published a study in 2005 in which he found that intensive lifestyle changes—including a completely plant-based diet—may affect the progression of early, low-grade prostate cancer in men. While more research is needed to confirm these findings and expand our understanding of them, studies like this one are a great reminder of the potential power our lifestyle choices may have.[7]

Recommendation 6: Alcoholic drinks

While the WCRF recommendation is to "limit alcoholic drinks," CHIP strongly recommends that the most appropriate advice is to abstain from or avoid alcohol. Aside from research showing links to cancer, alcohol has the potential for abuse, which can be devastating to the body and the mind. On top of this, alcohol is energy-dense, providing more calories per gram than any other nutrient except fat.

The WCRF states, "The evidence on cancer justifies a recommendation not to drink alcoholic drinks." The report continues: "The evidence does not show a clear level of consumption of alcoholic drinks below which there is no increase in risk of the cancers it causes." On its own, this is good reason to avoid alcohol consumption.

RED-WINE BENEFITS– WITHOUT THE ALCOHOL RISKS

While research surrounding red wine and possible benefits for heart health have received a lot of coverage in the media, research suggests that non-alcoholic red grape juice may also provide benefits to cardiovascular health. A study published in *Circulation*, the journal of the American Heart Association, investigated the effects of drinking purple grape juice on endothelial function and LDL cholesterol susceptibility to oxidations–a key process in the progression of atherosclerosis–in patients with coronary artery disease (CAD).

What the researchers found was that short-term ingestion of purple grape juice reduces LDL susceptibility to oxidation in CAD patients and improves the ability of major blood vessels to expand when blood flow increases. The researchers concluded that both of these are "potential mechanisms by which flavonoids in purple grape products may prevent cardiovascular events, independent of alcohol content."[8]

Remember, no one food is a magic cure. Grape juice may provide cardiovascular benefits, but remember it should still only be drunk in moderation, as it is an energy-dense drink.

Recommendation 7:
Preservation, processing, preparation

> Limit consumption of salt.

Personal Recommendations

> Avoid salt-preserved, salted or salty foods, and preserve foods without using salt.

> Limit consumption of processed foods with added salt to ensure an intake of less than 0.2 oz (6g) of salt—or 0.085 oz (2.4g) of sodium— per day.

The WCRF found on methods of food preservation, processing and preparation, that salt and salt-preserved foods were "probably a cause of stomach cancer" and foods contaminated with aflatoxins are a cause of liver cancer.

Low salt consumption has a number of benefits and is easy to achieve when consuming a diet of whole plant foods. Foods should be bought fresh and stored and prepared safely to get the maximum benefit.

Many canned vegetables are packed in salty brine, as a method of food preservation. But, perhaps surprisingly, not all canned foods contain the same amount of salt. Some canned vegetables, such as bean mixes, can be convenient foods to have in the cupboard for building quick, healthy meals. When choosing canned foods, compare products to find the lowest-salt version and rinse the foods well before using to wash off as much brine as possible.

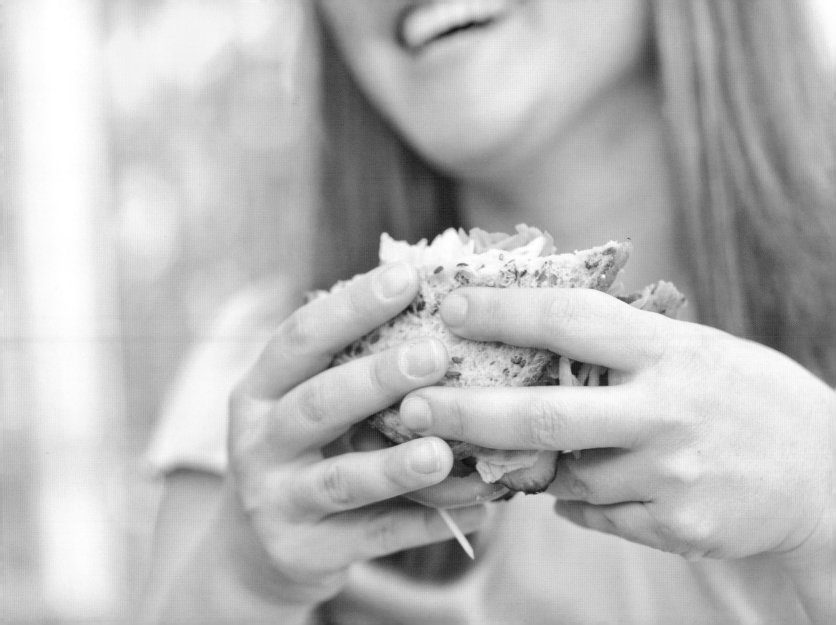

With the exception of vitamin B12, a completely plant-based diet can provide all the nutrients needed for an optimal lifestyle.

Recommendation 8: Dietary supplements

> Aim to meet nutritional needs through diet alone.

Personal Recommendation

> Dietary supplements are not recommended for cancer prevention.

The WCRF found that the evidence showed that, in certain circumstances, high-dose nutrient supplements can be protective against or can increase the risk of cancer. While dietary supplements may be needed in certain circumstances, they state high doses of vitamin supplements should not be used indiscriminately as "protection" against disease.

With the exception of vitamin B12, a completely plant-based diet can provide all the nutrients needed for an optimal lifestyle. In the case of vitamin B12, supplements are only recommended in required amounts, not in high dosages for "protective" benefits against disease.

When we consider these eight recommendations drawn from the leading cancer research available today, it should not surprise us that they include many of the aspects of lifestyle medicine we have been exploring in this book. Together, they are another reason why the optimal lifestyle—and all the everyday decisions that put it into practice in our lives—is key to optimal health.

> Cancer is an increasingly common disease that can affect many parts of the body.

> While research continues into cancer treatment and possible cure, research studies have identified significant risk factors for cancer development.

> The optimal lifestyle—including plant-based diet and active living—may reduce the risks of developing cancer in a number of important ways.

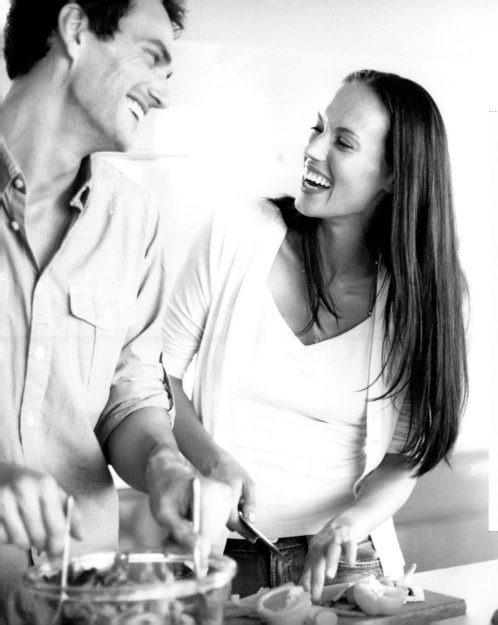

Chapter Eight References

1   Wiseman, M (2008), "The second World Cancer Research Fund/American Institute for Cancer Research expert report. Food, nutrition, physical activity, and the prevention of cancer: a global perspective," *Proceedings of the Nutrition Society,* Vol 67 No 3, pages 253-6.

2   World Health Organization (2012), "Cancer: fact sheet number 297."

3   Tao, M H, et al (2006), "Association of overweight with breast cancer survival," *American Journal of Epidemiology,* Vol 163 No 2, pages 101-7.

4   Pierce, J P, et al (2007), "Greater survival after breast cancer in physically active women with high vegetable-fruit intake regardless of obesity," *Journal of Clinical Oncology,* Vol 25 No 17, page 2345-51.

5   United States Department of Agriculture Nutrient Data Laboratory (2009)

6   Wu, A H, et al (2008), "Epidemiology of soy exposures and breast cancer risk," *British Journal of Cancer,* Vol 98 No 1, pages 9-14.

7   Ornish, D, et al (2005), "Intensive lifestyle changes may affect the progression of prostate cancer," *Journal of Urology,* Vol 174 No 3, pages 1065-9; discussion 1069-70.

8   Stein, J H, et al (1999), "Purple grape juice improves endothelial function and reduces the susceptibility of LDL cholesterol to oxidation in patients with coronary artery disease," *Circulation,* Vol 100 No 10, pages 1050-5.

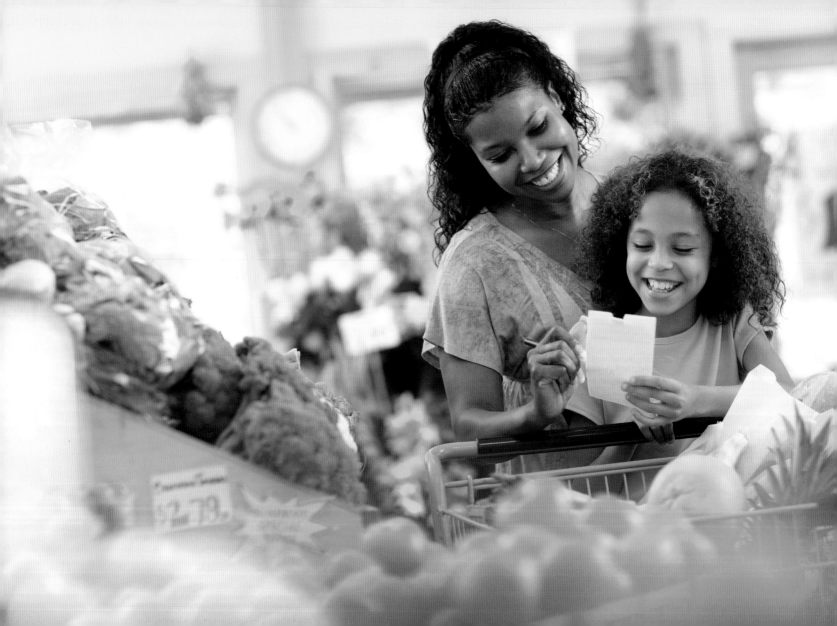

Chapter Nine

Nutritional Myth Busting

When it comes to the subject of health, there is no shortage of myths. It seems everyone has heard at least a handful of weird and wonderful remedies that are at best useless and at worst dangerous.

Nutrition is a particular area in which myths seem to take root and never let go. So let's explore three of the most common nutritional myths and shed some light into these dark corners of the food world.

MYTH: Dairy products must be consumed to maintain good bone health.

When you want to build a brick wall, obviously bricks are important. But bricks aren't anywhere near as useful without mortar to hold them together. Without mortar, you just have a pile of rocks. Alternatively, if you just used mortar without bricks, you'd have a pile of slowly drying mud. And if you have both and no skilled person assembling them properly, you'll still end up with a less than ideal result.

Strong bones are a lot like a brick wall. Science has identified a range of key building blocks for strong bones. On their own, these building blocks do not guarantee strength, but when used in the right amounts, put together properly and protected from things that could weaken them over time, they provide strength and good structure to help carry you through life.

Our bones are constantly rebuilding, with cells being replaced all the time. There are two main types of bone cells: osteoclasts that dissolve old bone cells; and osteoblasts that replace them and build up our bones. Imagine them as two laborers—one clearing away the old, worn wall, while the other busily lays bricks to replace it with a new one.

When this process works as intended, it helps produce strong bones. However, if osteoclast activity exceeds osteoblast activity or there are not enough materials available to build new bone, it can lead to weak, unhealthy bones.[1]

While about 99 per cent of calcium found in the body is stored in the bones and teeth, it is not stuck there. Bones act as a dynamic calcium bank, with calcium being withdrawn or deposited as needed by the body.[2]

› Calcium

When most people think about bone health, the first nutrient that comes to mind is calcium. While sufficient calcium in your diet is important for maintaining good bone health, it is not the only factor. Research shows that merely adding more and more calcium to the diet does not result in stronger bones.

If you ask the average person which foods are high in calcium, they will probably say dairy products. And they would be right: dairy products do contain high amounts of calcium. But much of the world's population suffer from lactose intolerance so cannot tolerate cow's milk or many other dairy products.[3] And, while dairy products are high in calcium, they can also be high in saturated fat, have no fiber and contain no protective phytonutrients. Research has shown those consuming a completely plant-based diet are at no greater risk of bone fracture than those who consume dairy products, if adequate calcium is consumed through other sources, which is not difficult to do.[4]

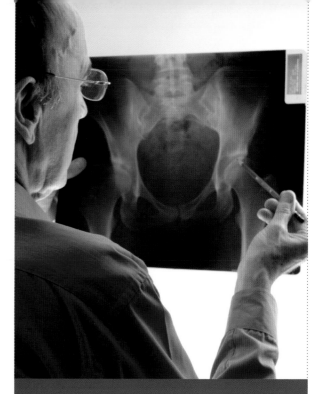

OSTEOPOROSIS

Osteoporosis is a condition in which bones slowly lose their strength, becoming weak and brittle, fracturing more easily. There is often no pain or obvious symptoms associated with the disease, so a fracture can be the first indication a person has of the disease. Osteoporosis appears more commonly in women in middle and later years, but can also affect men.

So how much calcium do we need?

Health organizations around the world give hugely different recommendations for calcium intake. In countries such as the United States and Canada, local health bodies recommend some of the highest calcium intakes in the world, while these countries also experience some of the highest rates of osteoporosis in the world.[5]

In its 2004 publication "Vitamin and mineral requirements in human nutrition," the World Health Organization recommends daily calcium intakes listed in this table (right):

However, the authors point out that these values were derived from studies in developed countries, acknowledging that these values are not applicable to everyone and that there are a number of factors that could lead to a person having increased requirements, including:

• Smoking,

• High salt intake, and

• Animal protein intake.

DAILY CALCIUM INTAKES RECOMMENDED BY WORLD HEALTH ORGANIZATION

	Recommended intake (mg/day)
Infants and children	
› *0-6 months*	
Human milk	*300*
Cow's milk	*400*
› *7-12 months*	*400*
› *1-3 years*	*500*
› *4-6 years*	*600*
› *7-9 years*	*700*
Adolescents	
› *10-18 years*	*1300*
Adults	
› Females	
19 years to menopause	*1000*
Postmenopause	*1300*
› Males	
19-65 years	*1000*
65+ years	*1300*
› Pregnant women (last trimester)	*1200*
› Lactating women	*1000*

While dairy products are high in calcium, they can also be high in saturated fat, have no fiber and contain no protective phytonutrients.

One such factor may be a high consumption of animal protein. Taking this into account, the authors put together theoretical calcium allowances based on an animal protein intake of 20-40g per day (representative of the animal protein intake of those in developing countries), rather than the 60-80g per day typical in developed countries, with theoretical daily requirements for some groups being as much as 500mg less!

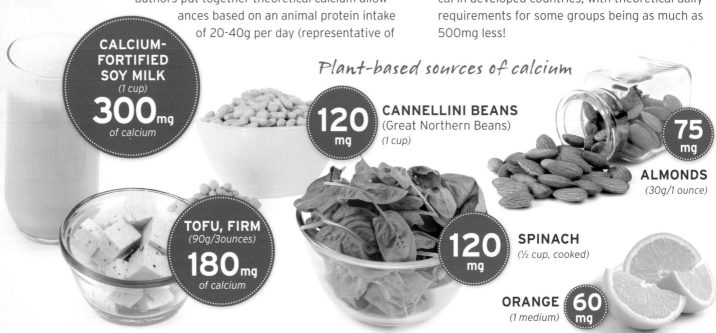

Plant-based sources of calcium

CALCIUM-FORTIFIED SOY MILK
(1 cup)
300mg of calcium

120 mg
CANNELLINI BEANS
(Great Northern Beans)
(1 cup)

75 mg
ALMONDS
(30g/1 ounce)

TOFU, FIRM
(90g/3ounces)
180mg of calcium

120 mg
SPINACH
(½ cup, cooked)

ORANGE
(1 medium)
60 mg

Bone health is not just about building up your bones, it's also about making sure they don't get torn down. Smoking, high salt intake[6] and soda/soft drinks have been linked with decreased bone health. Scientific modeling has shown that, theoretically, if a person's sodium intake was lowered from 3.45g per day to 1.15g, this could reduce their calcium requirement from 840mg to 600mg.[7]

› The sunshine vitamin

Another key to strong bones is vitamin D. It's a unique vitamin because we don't get the majority of what we need from our food, but from our skin being exposed to sunlight. Obtaining adequate vitamin D is a key component of good bone health. Worryingly, vitamin D deficiency appears to be a growing problem in many nations.[8]

How is vitamin D produced?

UVB rays in sunlight strike the skin and trigger the synthesis of vitamin D by first forming an inactive compound. This compound is taken to the liver, where changes occur, then to the kidneys where a final change converts it to usable vitamin D.[9] A few foods, such as oily fish and eggs, naturally contain vitamin D, which must also go through these activation steps in the body. While these foods contain vitamin D, the average person consumes only about 10 per cent of their daily need in this form, with sunlight being the most efficient way of meeting needs.[10]

But isn't too much time in the sun damaging?

Sun safety messages have been pushed heavily over the past few decades—and with good reason. Prolonged, unprotected sun exposure during peak UV times can be very damaging to the skin and a major risk factor for skin cancer. Check with your local health authority on their recommendations for safe sun exposure. Peak UV times can differ hugely from place to place and depending on the season.

Vitamin D synthesis doesn't mean sunbaking. In sunny parts of the world, particularly in summer, only about 10 to 15 minutes of sun exposure is needed to the hands, arms and face to produce significant amounts of vitamin D. Because of the way the body controls vitamin D production, short bursts of sun exposure are actually more effective than long bouts in the sun.

Only about 10 to 15 minutes of sun exposure is needed to the hands, arms and face to produce significant amounts of vitamin D.

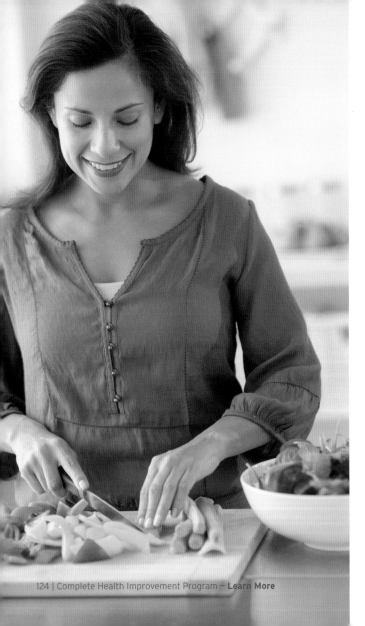

MYTH: You need to eat meat to get enough protein.

We live in a world that has an unhealthy obsession with protein. Protein is an important nutrient, and adequate amounts are needed to help support growth and repair in our bodies, but somewhere along the line we started consuming far more than is actually needed.

When we mention protein, most people think of meat but protein is also found in a wide range of plant foods, which are a much healthier package than their animal counterparts. In the more recent past, it was also believed that specific plant foods needed to be combined at meals for their protein to be useful. We now know that if a wide range of plant foods are consumed across the day, the body is quite capable of efficiently combining and using the protein they contain.[11]

› Protein requirements

More than a century ago, it was believed that we all needed at least 120g of protein daily.[12] The truth is we need much less than this and if enough calories are eaten as part of a varied plant-based diet, enough protein will also be consumed.[13]

Currently, the World Health Organization recommends a healthy adult aims for 0.83g of protein per 2.2 pounds (1 kg) of body weight.

165 LB (75 KG) MAN	130 LB (60 KG) WOMAN
62g protein per day	*50g protein per day*

What does adequate daily protein look like?

Consider this daily meal plan and the amount of protein it provides:

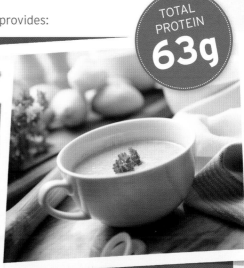

TOTAL PROTEIN 63g

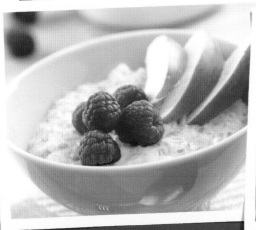

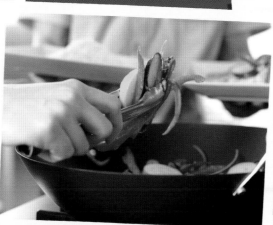

BREAKFAST	PROTEIN
› Porridge (1/2 cup rolled oats, 1 cup fat-free soy milk)	15.5g
› 2 teaspoons flaxseed	1g
› Fruit	1g

LUNCH	PROTEIN
› Vegetable stir-fry with tofu	14g
› Brown rice (1 cup)	6g
› Orange	1g

DINNER	PROTEIN
› Potato and leek soup	5.5g
› Fat-free soy milk (1 cup)	8g
› Whole wheat bread (2 slices)	5g
› Cashew nuts (small handful)	6g

Legumes—including beans, peas and lentils—are an amazing food group, packed full of nutrients and a good source of protein. Legumes are nutrition powerhouses, which should be included in the diet every day, making it even easier to meet protein needs on a plant-based diet.

Good plant-based sources of protein

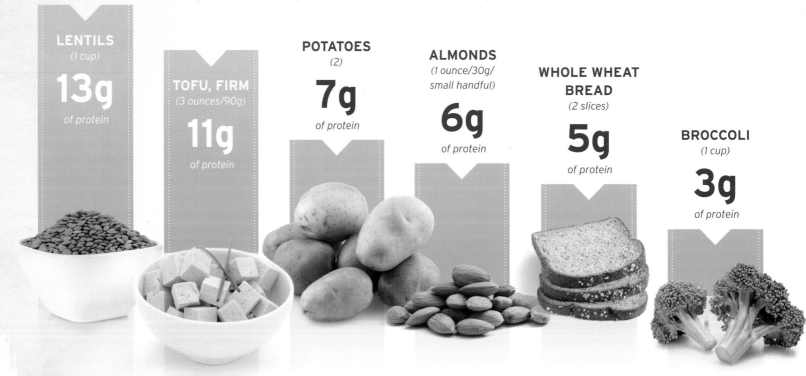

LENTILS
(1 cup)
13g
of protein

TOFU, FIRM
(3 ounces/90g)
11g
of protein

POTATOES
(2)
7g
of protein

ALMONDS
(1 ounce/30g/ small handful)
6g
of protein

WHOLE WHEAT BREAD
(2 slices)
5g
of protein

BROCCOLI
(1 cup)
3g
of protein

BRINGING THE RESEARCH TOGETHER

There are so many myths and misunderstandings about aspects of nutrition. When it comes to plant-based eating, there appear to be certain questions that are asked time and time again, despite there being much research to support not only the adequacy but also the healthfulness of plant-based eating. But wading through the published research—not to mention advertising, product labels, well-meaning advice from friends and family, news blogs and so on—and getting hold of credible sources can be tricky.

An Australian-first scientific review published in June, 2012, in the *Medical Journal of Australia* has answered a number of commonly held questions—and busted some common myths—about plant-based diets, some of which we have referenced in this chapter.

Does a plant-based diet provide enough protein? What about iron? And is it suitable for pregnant women? These and other questions are addressed in this excellent 40-page supplement, which provides evidence supporting the adequacy of plant-based diets. It shows that a well-planned plant-based diet can not only meet the nutritional needs of adults and children alike, but that it also reduces the risks of health problems such as cardiovascular disease, type 2 diabetes, high blood pressure and obesity.

The supplement also showcases sample meal plans across various life stages, as well as "Practical tips in Preparing Healthy and Delicious Plant-based Meals."

You can access this *Medical Journal of Australia* supplement at <www.mja.com.au/open/2012/1/2>.

For those seeking even more literature, we also recommend the 2012-published article "Health Implications of a Vegetarian Diet" by K Marsh, C Zeuschner and A Saunders.[14]

MYTH: You need to eat meat to get enough iron.

Much like protein, iron can be found in a wide range of foods we eat across the day, including plant-based foods. In fact, the type of iron found in plant based foods—non-haem iron or inorganic iron—is the main form of iron found in the average diet.[15]

The recommended daily dietary intakes of iron range from 8 to 18mg, depending on age and gender, and is higher for women during pregnancy.[16]

Iron-rich plant foods[17]
Per 3.5oz (100g)

CURLY LEAF PARSLEY	11.5mg
IRON-FORTIFIED WHOLE WHEAT CEREAL	10.5mg
TEMPEH	9.2mg
CASHEWS	6.3mg
SUNDRIED TOMATOES	5.6mg
MIXED GRAIN BREAD ROLL	5.6mg
PINE NUTS	4.1mg
ALMONDS (with skins)	3.9mg
ENGLISH SPINACH	3.9mg
DRIED APRICOTS	3.3mg
TOFU (firm)	2.9mg
SILVER BEET (boiled)	2.8mg
DRIED DATES	2.6mg
PEANUTS	2.4mg
SOY BEANS, KIDNEY BEANS AND LENTILS	2.0-2.2mg
SULTANAS	2.0mg
GREEN PEAS/BAKED BEANS	1.7mg

Non-haem iron is not as readily absorbed as that found in animal foods. But research has confirmed that vegetarians who eat a varied and well-balanced diet—including whole grains, legumes, nuts, seeds, dried fruits, iron-fortified cereals and green leafy vegetables—are not at any greater risk of iron deficiency than non-vegetarians.[18]

A few simple tips can help maximize the absorption of iron from the plant-based diet:

> **Include a good source of vitamin C with your plant-based sources of iron.** Vitamin C helps facilitate the absorption of plant-based iron. Vitamin C can be found in foods such as citrus fruits, tomatoes and bell peppers (capsicum).

> **Avoid tea, coffee and cola drinks, particularly with meals.** These drinks contain compounds that can bind to iron and prevent it from being absorbed efficiently.

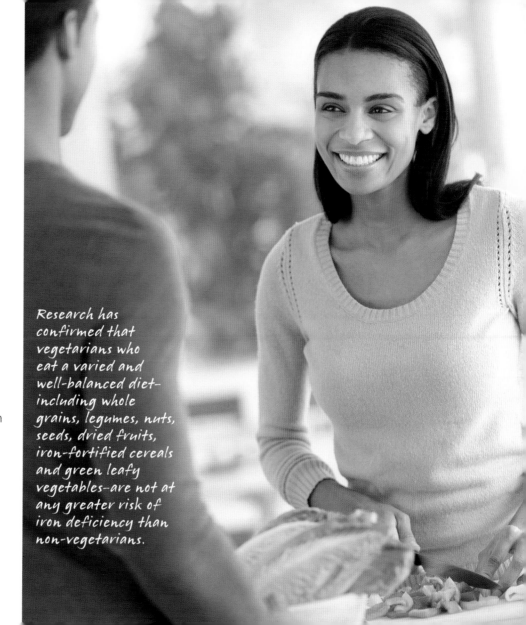

Research has confirmed that vegetarians who eat a varied and well-balanced diet—including whole grains, legumes, nuts, seeds, dried fruits, iron-fortified cereals and green leafy vegetables—are not at any greater risk of iron deficiency than non-vegetarians.

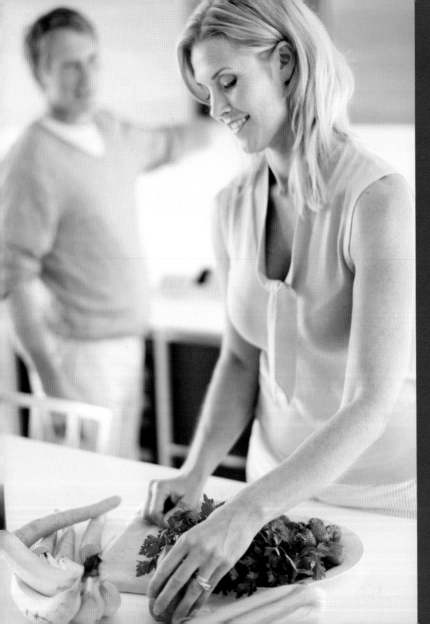

BE SMART ABOUT B12

Vitamin B12 is an essential water-soluble vitamin that plays a key role in the proper functioning of the brain and nervous system. It is also important for development of the brain and nervous system, so is vital for women during pregnancy and breast feeding. You may have heard that it is an animal-based vitamin, because we find most of it in meat and other animal products, but vitamin B12 is actually produced by bacteria and microorganisms that live in those animals, in our environment and also in us.

While we need only a small amount daily, it is important that we meet those requirements and we don't get enough from our own bacteria, nor from the plant foods we eat. In the past, it was believed that mushrooms contained usable vitamin B12, but we now know this is not the case. So if you choose to opt for a 100 per cent plant-based diet for all its amazing health benefits, where are you going to get your vitamin B12 from?

The good news is that many vegetarian foods, such as soy milk, come fortified with vitamin B12 (check the label) and supplements are available to help meet daily needs, without having to include animal foods in the diet. Today, we have so many easy and affordable options available.

Vitamin B12 deficiency can take some time to show symptoms, sometimes even years, so discuss your vitamin B12 needs with your doctor, who can check your levels to help ensure you are not deficient, especially if you are pregnant or breastfeeding.

Chapter Nine References

1. Boyce, B F, Z Yao, and L Xing (2009), "Osteoclasts have multiple roles in bone in addition to bone resorption," *Critical Reviews in Eukaryot Gene Expression*, Vol 19 No 3, page 171-80.

2. Ross, A C, and Institute of Medicine (US) (2011), "Dietary reference intakes : calcium, vitamin D," *Committee to Review Dietary Reference Intakes for Vitamin D and Calcium*, National Academies Press, xv, 536, page 1115.

3. Scrimshaw, N S and E B Murray (1988), "The acceptability of milk and milk products in populations with a high prevalence of lactose intolerance," *American Journal of Clinical Nutrition*, Vol 48 No 4 Supplement, pages 1079-159.

4. Appleby, P, et al (2007), "Comparative fracture risk in vegetarians and nonvegetarians in EPIC-Oxford," *European Journal of Clinical Nutrition*, Vol 61 No 12, pages 1400-6.

5. World Health Organization. and Food and Agriculture Organization of the United Nations (2004), *Vitamin and mineral requirements in human nutrition* (2nd ed), World Health Organization, FAO xix.

6. Walser, M (161), "Calcium clearance as a function of sodium clearance in the dog," *American Journal of Physiology*, Vol 200, pages 1099-104; Sabto, J, et al (1984), "Influence of urinary sodium on calcium excretion in normal individuals. A redefinition of hypercalciuria," *Medical Journal of Australia*, Vol 140 No 6, pages 354-6.

7. WHO, op cit.

8. Mithal, A, et al (2009), "Global vitamin D status and determinants of hypovitaminosis D," *Osteoporosis International*, Vol 20 No 11, pages 1807-20.

9. Institute of Medicine, F a N B (2010), *Dietary Reference Intakes for Calcium and Vitamin D*, National Academy Press; Cranney, A, et al (2007), "Effectiveness and safety of vitamin D in relation to bone health," *Evidence Report/Technology Assessment* (Full Report), Vol 158, pages 1-235.

10. Mithal, op cit.

11. American Dietetic Association and Dietitians of Canada (2003), "Position of the American Dietetic Association and Dietitians of Canada: vegetarian diets," *Canadian Journal of Dietetic Practice and Research*, Vol 64 No 2, pages 62-81.

12. Chittenden, R H (1904), *Physiological economy in nutrition, with special reference to the minimal protein requirement of the healthy man*, F A Stokes Co.

13. Marsh, K A, et al (2012), "Protein and Vegetarian Diets," *Medical Journal of Australia Open*, Vol 1 Supplement 2, pages 7-10.

14. Marsh, K, C Zeuschner and A Saunders (2012), "Health Implications of a Vegetarian Diet: A Review," *American Journal of Lifestyle Medicine*, Vol 6 No 4, pages 250-67.

15. WHO, op cit.

16. National Health and Medical Research Council and New Zealand Ministry of Health (2006), *Nutrient reference values for Australia and New Zealand including recommended dietary intakes*, NHMRC.

17. Food Standards Australia New Zealand, *NUTTAB 2006*, <www.foodstandards.gov.au/consumerinformation/nuttab2006/>.

18. Saunders, A V, et al (2012), "Iron and vegetarian diets," *Medical Journal of Australia Open*, Vol 1 Supplement 2, pages 11-16.

Section 3

The Optimal Active Lifestyle

In the field of lifestyle medicine, physical activity is recognized as one of the key pillars of health and healing. In this section, we consider the merits of this great panacea and why it is becoming increasingly imperative that we move more.

Chapter Ten explores the reasons we have become increasingly sedentary over the past century and the associated perils from a health and wellbeing perspective. On a positive note, it also highlights the benefits of an active lifestyle.

Chapter Eleven details the ingredients of the optimal active lifestyle, which includes being intentional about sitting less and moving more throughout the day, engaging in regular "aerobic" exercise, and performing exercises that develop strength and suppleness.

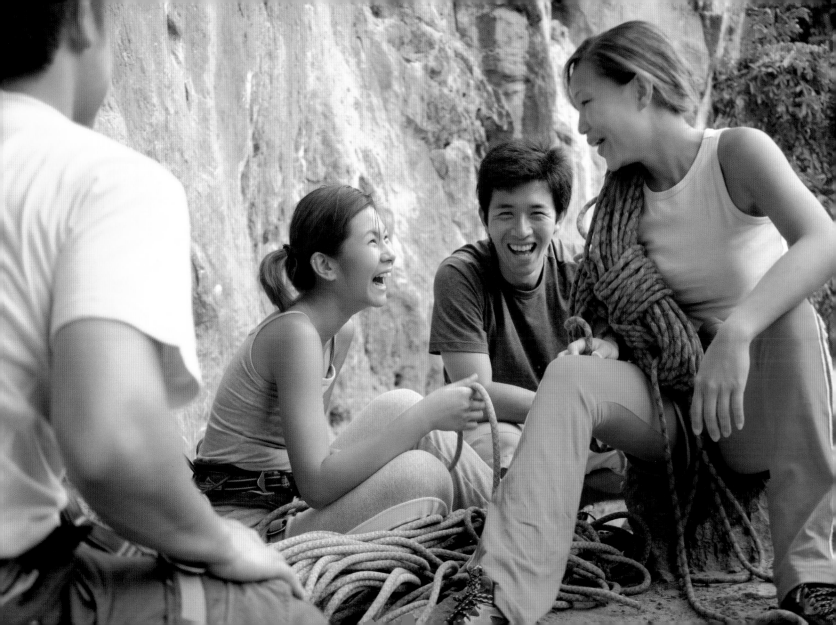

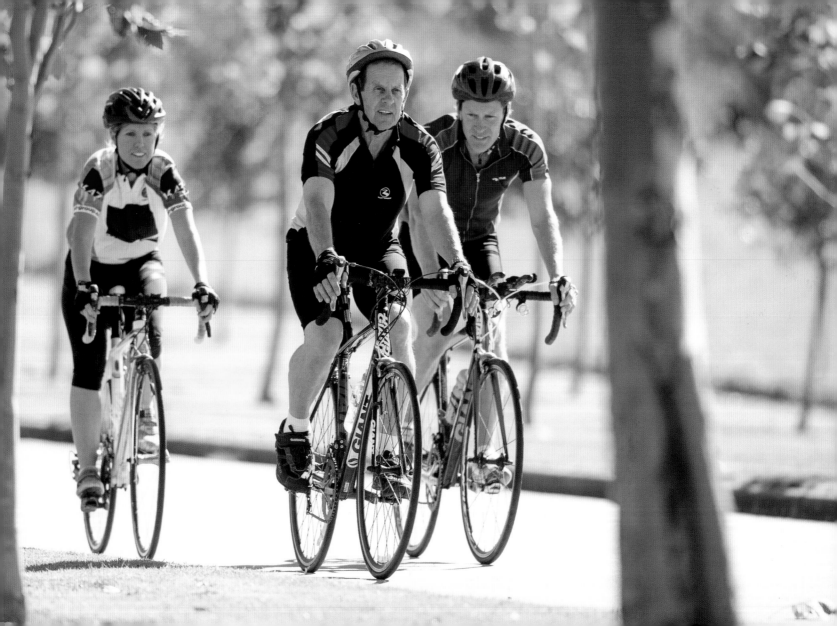

Chapter Ten

Made to Move!

It has been estimated that in developed countries, we are 60 to 70 per cent less active than a century ago, which equates to walking about 10 miles (about 16 kilometers) less each day.[1] Furthermore, as illustrated, most of this decline has occurred in the past 40 years. Several factors have contributed to this but largely to blame is the advent of "modern conveniences" that allow us to expend less energy doing our daily tasks.

As a society, we have been carried away with inventing movement-saving devices. We have ingeniously created devices that wash the dishes for us, deliver warm water straight to our bath so we don't have to walk or work to get it, lift us higher in a building bypassing the stairs, and change the channel on our television with the press of a remote button so we don't have to get out of our seat.

While there are many benefits and much to enjoy in our modern technology and labor-saving devices, we have created an environment in which being inactive has never been easier. Our innovative technologies have especially changed the nature of our work, transportation and recreation—and that is a problem because we are made to move.

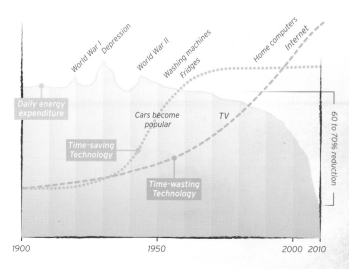

The changing patterns of physical activity in industrialized countries over the 20th Century.[2]

Work

In the 1950s, Dr Jerry Morris first documented the dangers of inactivity in a study of more than 30,000 London bus service employees.[3] According to Dr Morris, the bus drivers—who sat in their comfortable seats all day long—were about three times more likely to die from a heart attack than the conductors who were on their feet all day. Dr Morris also noted that the average uniform size of the drivers was larger than the uniforms of the conductors, suggesting a link between inactivity, obesity and heart health. Since that time, the work of most individuals has become increasingly inactive. Fewer and fewer people arrive at work on Monday morning anticipating a day of heavy physical labor. Instead, an increasing number sit in front of a computer screen.

Transportation

One hundred years ago, lengthy travel time would not have been a problem because it would have required us to use our legs. But today we get places by sitting—in the car, bus, train or plane. Furthermore, the length of time we spend in transportation has increased substantially with urbanization. An increasing number of individuals are forced to commute long distances to get from the suburbs where they live to the city where they work. It is not uncommon in large cities for individuals to travel up to two hours to work, then another two hours home. When added to the eight or more hours sitting at work, this represents a huge portion of the day spent inactive.

Recreation

The invention of television revolutionized the way people spent their free time and the development of the internet and computer-based entertainment has further increased the time we are inactive. Indeed, "screen time" is a major contributor to our sedentary lifestyles. Unlike the 1950s when only about 10 per cent of homes had a television set,[4] today almost every home has at least one. Similarly, the number of homes with internet access has skyrocketed since the late 1990s. Unfortunately, it is not just adults who are glued to the screens: children are also spending far too much time playing video games, communicating with their friends over the internet or watching television. Alarmed by the amount of screen time children are experiencing, peak health bodies encourage parents to limit their children's screen time to not more than two hours per day.

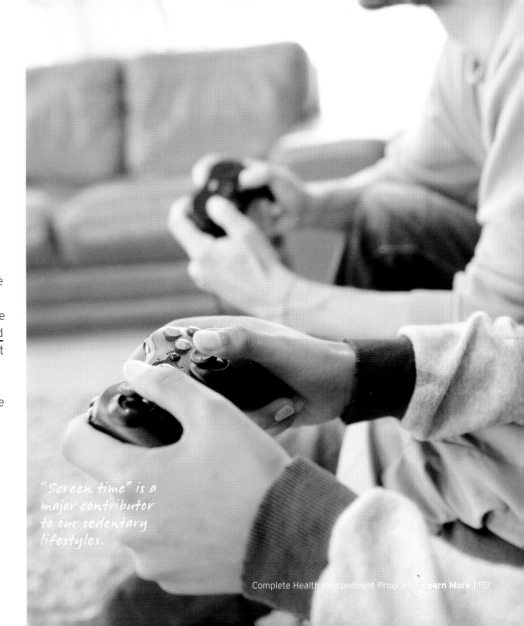

"Screen time" is a major contributor to our sedentary lifestyles.

Why be active?

Clearly we are far less active than previous generations, but does that matter? Research is demonstrating that it matters a lot. The human body is designed to be active and when it is not operated according to its design, things go wrong. Indeed, inactivity brings with it much bad news, but the good news is that increasing your levels of physical activity can do tremendous good.

› More life

Inactivity increases your risk of dying young, whereas being physically active extends your life. More than 30 years ago, it was first observed that champion male Finnish skiers lived on average 4.1 years longer than "average" Finnish men.[5] Since that time, it has become clear that former elite athletes tend to live longer than us mere mortals. But you don't have to be an Olympian to look forward to a long life.

An investigation of the longest-living people on earth—the Okinawans, Sardinians and Seventh-day Adventists—showed one of the things they all have in common is they "moved naturally."[6] In other words, they engaged in plenty of physical activity as part of their daily living.

A concentrated study of the Seventh-day Adventist community—the famous "Adventist Health Study"—identified being physically active as one of five key lifestyle choices. This research found that physical activity, along with not smoking, eating nuts regularly, being vegetarian, and maintaining a healthy body weight, could add as many as 10 years to your life, with each of these recommended lifestyle choices adding between 1.5 and 2.5 years of life expectancy.[7]

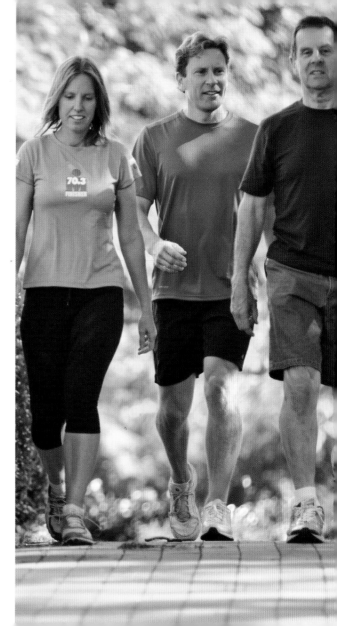

› More vibrant life

Inactivity kills vitality, whereas regular physical activity makes you feel more energetic and vibrant. The oft-repeated joke about healthy living asks, "If I make positive lifestyle changes and kick the bad habits, will I live longer or will it just feel longer?" But while regular physical activity can add years to your life, it also adds life to your years. Being physically active boosts vitality in a number of ways.

First, it increases your energy levels. It is a strange reality that by regularly expending energy—by being physically active—we get more!

Second, regular physical activity makes you feel better by stimulating the release of mood-enhancing chemicals in your brain, referred to as endorphins. Incredibly, endorphins have similar effects to opiate drugs in that they reduce pain and make you feel euphoric. Unlike opiate drugs, however, they are good for you. In fact, there is increasing evidence that exercise is good for your brain in many ways, and enhances cognitive and brain function.[8]

The ability of regular physical activity to positively influence brain chemistry and elevate mood is one of the reasons exercise is key for the management of depression. Physical activity can also burn up stress hormones that keep us awake at night, so it can help improve sleep quality. Living in a constant state of sleep deprivation as a result of poor quality sleep will make anyone feel lousy—and those who have to live with them—so this is another way physical activity can help elevate our feelings of vitality.

Third, regular physical activity not only makes you feel good in yourself, it also makes you feel good *about* yourself. Studies have shown that regular physical activity improves an individual's perception of their physical condition and body attractiveness and increases their sense of self-worth.

Regular physical activity not only makes you feel good in yourself, it also makes you feel good about yourself.

› Protection against disease

Being physically active protects against the development of numerous diseases, while inactivity is linked to numerous adverse diseases and conditions including:[9]

› Coronary heart disease
› Stroke
› High blood pressure
› High cholesterol
› Type 2 diabetes
› Osteoporosis
› Colon cancer
› Breast cancer
› Lung cancer
› Endometrial cancer

Being physically active can not only help prevent these conditions, it can also help manage some of them. In a study comparing the effectiveness of exercise training with the surgical procedure of stenting in patients with stable coronary heart disease, exercise was found to be superior in avoiding re-hospitalizations and re-vascularization procedures, and it also resulted in better survival rates.[10] Exercise is also now seen to be as important as nutritional prescription for type 2 diabetes.[11]

Clearly there are many health benefits associated with maintaining an active lifestyle. The extent to which regular activity positively influences our health, and the mechanisms by which it does, are becoming more fully understood. Exercise has long been known to decrease blood pressure, improve cholesterol status and "flush" the body of toxins, but it is now also known to increase the production of *antioxidants* that neutralize free radicals, the damaging agents that arise in the body.[12] As free radicals contribute to the progression of many diseases, the capacity of exercise to help the body combat them may in part also explain exercise's health-promoting qualities. Moderate physical activity is also known to boost the body's immune system.

If you could develop a pill that packaged the benefits that come from regular physical activity, it would be a major medical breakthrough. You would get rich quick as everyone would want to swallow it. The great news is that physical activity is the cure everyone can take—and it's free! Appropriately, many peak exercise bodies including the American College of Sports Medicine and Exercise and Sports Science Australia have adopted the catch cry, *"Exercise is Medicine."*

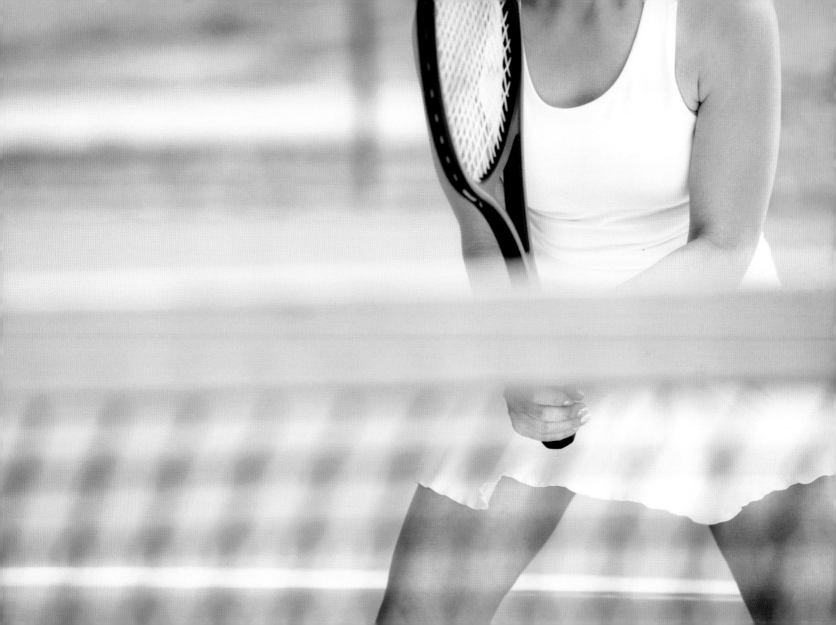

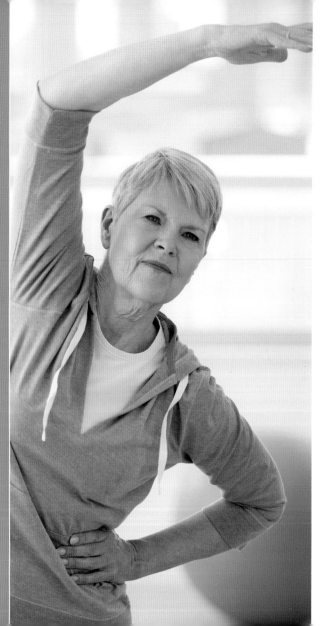

ADDED BENEFITS

Some of the additional benefits of keeping active include:

> Improved weight loss and prevention of weight gain

> Improved cognitive function

> Stronger bones, resulting in prevention of falls

> Improved functional health (especially for older adults)

> Reduced depression

› Live stronger

Inactivity decreases our strength and physical function, whereas regular physical activity makes us stronger and more functional. As we grow older, strength and stability become increasingly important. Performing strength-building exercises can powerfully improve muscular strength and greatly enhance daily functioning as a result. For older adults, this can make the difference between independent living or having to rely on others. But strength-building exercises not only increase muscular strength, they also increase the strength of the bones to which the muscles are attached.

› Live leaner

Inactivity promotes weight gain, whereas physical activity promotes weight loss. Worldwide, obesity has more than doubled since 1980, and today 65 per cent of the world's population live in countries where more people die as a result of being overweight than being underweight.[13] While genetics are often blamed for the obesity epidemic, genetics clearly don't explain the overwhelming increase in obesity over the past 30 years. The human genome has not changed significantly in that time. The amount genetics contribute to obesity is a topic of debate but one thing is for sure: no-one gets fat if they don't eat or if they are sufficiently active.

Numerous studies point to regular physical activity being an integral part of the solution to the obesity epidemic, especially for keeping lost weight off. An expert report by the World Cancer Research Fund gave their highest commendation—"convincing"—to the role exercise plays in managing obesity.[14] This is not to discount the importance of diet in effective weight management, but it does highlight that physical activity is an equally important pillar of weight control.

One reason that exercise can be more effective than dieting for long-term weight loss is because once we get in the swing of exercising, our body craves it. This occurs because the opiate-like endorphins produced in response to exercise not only make you feel better, they are also addictive. This is why regular exercisers have withdrawal-type symptoms if they can't be active when they usually would be.

Exercise, therefore, becomes a self-perpetuating behavior. By contrast, we never lose the drive to want to eat—hunger is a deeply ingrained, innate drive that prevents us from starving to death. It is almost impossible to go through life hungry and calorie restrictive diets are unsustainable in the long-term as a result.

EXERCISE AND APPETITE

Does exercise increase appetite and therefore cause you to eat more? The answer seems to be both "yes" and "no."

Exercise does seem to increase appetite in people who are of a healthy weight. This is hardly surprising given that someone who is not carrying extra energy reserves—also known as, body fat—needs to replace the energy used during exercise from somewhere! Exercise doesn't however seem to cause the same increase in appetite in overweight individuals—it can actually decrease their feelings of hunger.[15]

Essentially, exercise seems to help with appetite regulation. It helps our brain get better at deciding how much energy our body actually needs, then adjusts our desire to eat accordingly.[16]

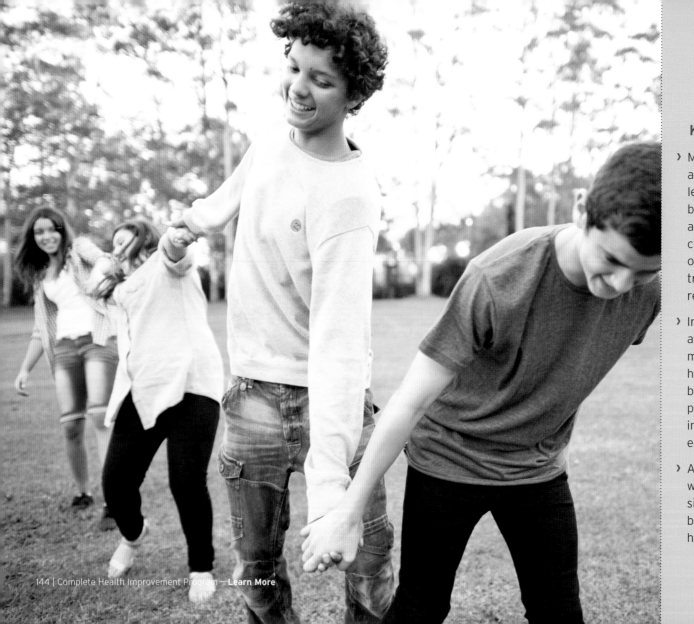

KEY POINTS

› Many of us are moving less than ever before, largely as a result of the changing nature of our work, transportation and recreation.

› Inactivity is associated with many adverse health outcomes but becoming physically active is incredibly health enhancing.

› A daily 30-minute walk can bring significant positive benefits to our health.

Made to move

We are made to move—but unfortunately we are not doing enough of it. This is resulting in many undesirable outcomes in terms of our health and wellbeing. As such, Professor Stephen Blair of the Aerobic Centre Longitudinal Study has said, "Evidence supports the conclusion that physical inactivity is one of the most important public health problems of the 21st century, and may even be the most important."[17]

The good news is that embracing an active lifestyle can prevent, and in some cases even reverse, many of the ills that presently plague developed countries. Our journey to health begins with a single step—and then another.

Chapter Ten References

1   Vogels, N, et al (2004), "Estimating Changes in Daily Physical Activity Levels over Time: Implication for Health Interventions from a Novel Approach," *International Journal of Sports Medicine*, Vol 25, pages 607-10.

2   ibid.

3   Morris, J N, et al (1953), "Coronary heart disease and physical activity of work," *The Lancet*, Vol 2, pages 1111-20.

4   Brownson, R C, T K Boehmer and D A Luke (2005), "Declining rate of physical activity in the US: what are the contributors?" *Annual Review of Public Health*, Vol 26, pages 421-43.

5   Karvonen, M J (1976), "Sports and Longevity," *Advances in Cardiology*, Vol 18, pages 243-8.

6   Buettner, D (2008), *The Blue Zones: Lessons for living longer from the people who have lived the longest*, National Geographic Society, Washington, page 231.

7   Fraser, G E, and D J Shavlik (2001), "Ten years of life: is it a matter of choice?" *Archive of Internal Medicine*, Vol 161, pages 1645-52.

8   Kraemer, A F, and K I Erickson (2007), "Capitalizing on cortical plasticity: influence of PA on cognition and gut function," *Trends in Cognitive Science*, Vol 11 No 8, pages 342-8.

9   2008 Physical Activity Guidelines for Americans, <www.health.gov/paguidelines>.

10 Hambrecht, C W, et al (2004), "Percutaneous Coronary Angioplasty Compared With Exercise Training in Patients With Stable Coronary Artery Disease : A Randomized Trial," *Circulation*, Vol 109, pages 1371-8.

11 Egger G, Binns A, Rossner S (2011), *Lifestyle Medicine—Managing diseases of lifestyle in the 21st century*, McGraw-Hill Australia Pty Ltd, page 115.

12 Mathur, H, and B K Pedersen (2008), "Exercise as a Means to Control Low-Grade Systemic Inflammation," *Mediators of Inflammation*, Volume 2008, Article ID 109502.

13 World Health Organization, <www.who.int/mediacentre/factsheets/fs311/en/>, accessed April, 2012.

14 World Cancer Research Fund, (2007), "Food, Nutrition, Physical Activity, and the prevention of cancer: a global perspective," *American Institute of Cancer Research*.

15 Martins, C, et al (2008), "A review of the effects of exercise on appetite regulation: an obesity perspective," *International Journal of Obesity*, Vol 32, pages 1337-47.

16 Martins, C, et al (2010), "The Effects of Exercise-Induced Weight Loss on Appetite-Related Peptides and Motivation to Eat," *Journal of Clinical Endocrinology and Metabolism*, Vol 95 No 4, pages 1609-16.

17 Blair, S (2009), "Physical inactivity: the biggest public health problem of the 21st century," *British Journal of Sports Medicine*, Vol 43 No 1, pages 1-2.

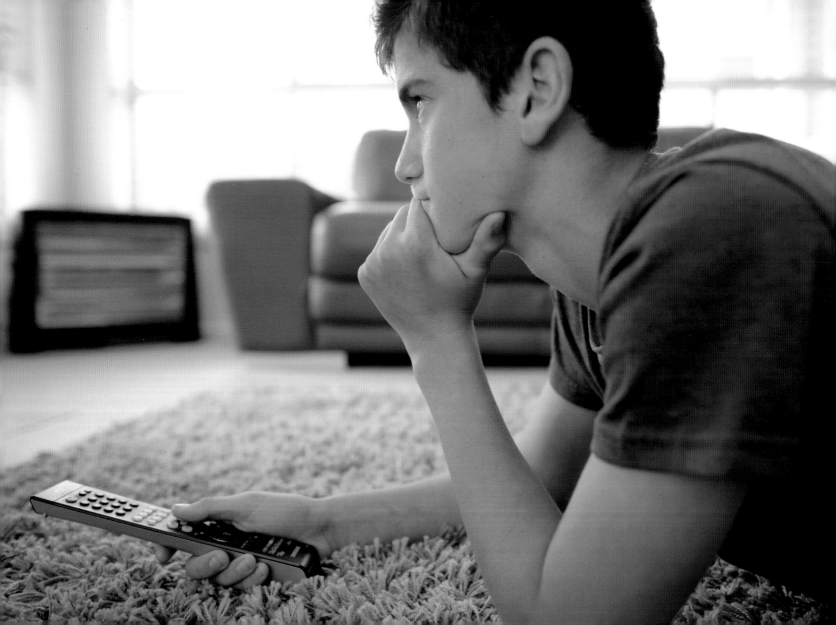

Chapter Eleven

Step into Active Living

We live in an environment geared toward inactivity, so it is little wonder that our default is to be underactive. For centuries, we simply *were* active but today we need to be intentional about moving more, if we are to achieve the levels of activity our bodies need to thrive.

STEP 1: Less sitting, more moving!

We are discovering that the long-term ill-health consequences of too much sitting and not enough moving during the day are distinct from the consequences of not exercising. In other words, while exercising daily has many health-promoting benefits, if you spend the rest of your day sitting around and not moving, your risk of ill-health, disease and premature death jumps back up!

In a study of more than 120,000 adults monitored for 14 years, people who sat for extended periods in their leisure time and did not exercise had a greatly increased risk of premature death—a 94 per cent increase for women and a 48 per cent increase for men.[1] At first there appeared to be nothing surprising about these results, as it simply demonstrated the well-established importance of being physically active on our health. But as the researchers more thoroughly mined the data, they noticed a fascinating trend. Those individuals who exercised regularly but then sat for extended periods during the day still had a greatly increased death rate—as much as a 40 per cent higher rate for women and 20 per cent for men.

In another study, after precluding most of the recognized risk factors for disease, individuals

We are discovering that the long-term ill-health consequences of too much sitting . . . are distinct from the consequences of not exercising.

ACCUMULATED SIT TIME OF AN "ACTIVE COUCH POTATO"[2]

WATCHING TV, READING
4 hours

SLEEP
8 hours

EAT DINNER
30 minutes

STRENGTH TRAINING
30 minutes

DRIVE HOME
1 hour

BRISK WALK
30 minutes

DRIVE TO WORK
1 hour

WORK ON COMPUTER
4 hours

WORK ON COMPUTER
4 hours

LUNCH
30 minutes

who engaged in more than four hours of screen-based entertainment per day had a 48 per cent increased chance of dying from all-causes and a 125 per cent increased likelihood of suffering a cardiovascular event.[3]

The problem is that we live in a society in which sitting is the default. As pictured left, it is easy to accumulate 15 hours of sit time in a day, despite this individual being diligent enough to perform 60 minutes of exercise, far beyond the achievements of most of us! Such individuals are described as "active couch potatoes."

The dangers of prolonged sitting are becoming so apparent that a new field of study—"inactivity physiology"—is emerging. Researchers in this field have discovered that prolonged periods of sitting and not moving alter the body's control over cholesterol in a negative way—especially the bad LDL cholesterol—and places individuals at increased risk of cardiovascular disease.[4]

But it is not just the amount of sedentary time we accumulate, it is how it is accumulated. Prolonged uninterrupted sit time appears to be the real danger. Regularly breaking up periods of sitting with short periods of movement—even just standing every 30 minutes—is associated with lower measures of waist circumference, body mass index, blood triglycerides and fasting plasma glucose levels.[5]

The message is that most of us are sitting far too much in an uninterrupted fashion—and it is to our detriment. The solution is apparent—don't just sit there! No longer can we afford to think of *having* to move as a time-wasting bother. Instead, we need to start thinking of it as an opportunity to invest in our own health and wellbeing. Every bit counts—and it begins with less sitting and more moving.

PRACTICAL TIPS FOR LESS SIT TIME[6]

At home

> Move around the house when talking on the telephone.
> Take the batteries out of the TV remote control so you have to get out of your seat to change channels.
> Stand up and walk around the house during TV commercial breaks.
> Do household chores that involve standing, such as ironing, while watching TV.
> Stand to read the morning newspaper.

At work

> Stand and take a break from your computer every 30 minutes.
> Stand periodically during long meetings. (Explain what you are doing at the start and you might encourage others to do likewise.)
> Stand to greet a visitor to your worksite.
> Stand during phone calls.
> Take the stairs.
> Drink more water so that you have to go fetch it and visit the bathroom more often.
> Move items such as your rubbish bin, filing cabinet and printer further away, so you are forced to get out of your seat to use them.
> Use a height-adjustable desk, so you can alternate between sitting and standing.
> Organize standing or "walk while we talk" meetings instead of the usual sit-a-thons. Your brain will work better, too!
> Stand at the back of the room during presentations.
> Eat your lunch away from your desk.

When travelling

> Park your car further away from your destination and walk the rest of the way.
> Plan regular breaks during long car trips.
> Use public transport so you have to walk to and from stops or stations.
> Get on or off public transport one stop or station before your destination and walk the rest of the way.
> On public transport, offer your seat to someone who needs it.

STEP 2: Breathe more

For many people, the word "exercise" conjures up images of pain and discomfort. Since our brains are motivated to avoid pain, it is little wonder so many people avoid exercise or at least think of it as something to be endured, rather than enjoyed. But exercise need not be painful for us to experience great benefits. There is no truth to the popular saying, "No pain, no gain."

While there are great benefits for those who sit less and move more throughout the day, far greater rewards come to those who engage in regular physical activity that causes an increased breathing rate. Activities that cause us to breathe more—like brisk walking, swimming, cycling and jogging—are referred to as "aerobic" exercises.

› Get thrilled about 30!

Aerobic exercise was first popularized more than 40 years ago by Dr Kenneth Cooper, who began to research its effect on health and wellbeing. Dr Cooper's research has grown into the world-leading Aerobic Center Longitudinal Study, which now involves more than 250,000 records from almost 100,000 individuals. This study has shown that individuals who participate in around 150 minutes of moderate-intensity aerobic exercise each week—about 30 minutes most days—have a greatly reduced risk of premature death.

Many countries have developed physical activity guidelines consistent with these recommendations. Further research indicates that the 30 minutes can be broken down into three 10-minute blocks that can be spread throughout the day.[7] This is good news for individuals who struggle to find a solid 30-minute space in their day.

Moderate-intensity exercise: Such exercise causes a noticeable increase in breathing rate but you can still maintain an uninterrupted conversation. Such intensity could be maintained for 30 to 60 minutes and would rate as an effort of 3-or-4-out-of-10.[8] Examples of moderate-intensity physical activity might include: gentle swimming, social tennis, walking with a purpose or cycling at a regular pace. Clearly, moderate-intensity exercise is not pain-evoking and is achievable for most of us.

THE RISK OF DYING PREMATURELY DECLINES AS PEOPLE ENGAGE IN MORE AEROBIC EXERCISE

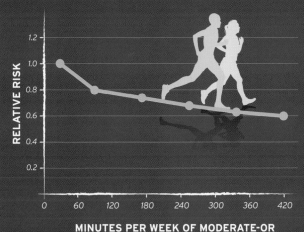

MINUTES PER WEEK OF MODERATE-OR VIGOROUS-INTENSITY PHYSICAL ACTIVITY

The Aerobic Center Longitudinal Study has shown that individuals who participate in around 150 minutes of moderate-intensity aerobic exercise each week—about 30 minutes most days—have a greatly reduced risk of premature death.

Examples of EXERCISE

Moderate-intensity physical activity includes:

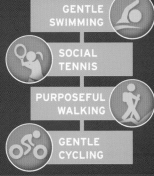

GENTLE SWIMMING

SOCIAL TENNIS

PURPOSEFUL WALKING

GENTLE CYCLING

Vigorous-intensity physical activity includes:

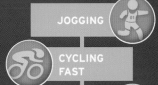

JOGGING

CYCLING FAST

AEROBIC CLASSES

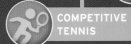

COMPETITIVE TENNIS

Vigorous-intensity exercise: For those who enjoy pushing harder and are capable of doing so, the guidelines suggest extra benefits can be achieved through vigorous-intensity exercise. Vigorous-intensity physical activity describes exercise during which a conversation could not be maintained uninterrupted—you would need to catch your breath between sentences. The intensity could usually not be sustained for more than 30 minutes at a time and it would rate as a 5-or-6-out-of-10 effort.[9] Vigorous-intensity physical activity might include: jogging, cycling fast, aerobic classes and competitive tennis.

Intensity of effort is relative to your fitness level. For example, jogging at a certain pace might be impossible for one individual and therefore described as beyond "vigorous," while another individual might glide along effortlessly at that same speed and the intensity would be judged "moderate" or even "light." It is important that you get to know what constitutes moderate and vigorous intensity for you.

As you are walking or performing different physical activities, get into the habit of asking yourself, "What would I rate this effort out of 10?"

If it is a 3 to 4, then it is moderate-intensity, while a 5 or above is entering the realm of vigorous. There are other methods for judging how taxing a certain exercise level is on your body by using devices such as a heart rate monitor, but unless you are training for high-level fitness, subjectively gauging your own level of intensity is sufficient.

If you are concerned that exercise might be dangerous as it can bring on heart attacks, consider the following statistics. Estimates of sudden cardiac death rates during exercise range from 0 to 2 per 100,000 exercise hours in the general population and from 0.13 to 0.61 per 100,000 exercise hours in cardiac rehabilitation programs.[10] While it is good to get the all-clear from your doctor before getting serious with an exercise program, the benefits clearly outweigh the risks.

OVERWEIGHT BUT FIT?

While aerobic exercise is extremely helpful for managing body weight, research has demonstrated that it offers health benefits independent of weight loss. In other words, it is possible to be overweight but also fit and that fitness will ameliorate many of the health hazards of obesity.[11] Indeed, obese individuals who are active have lower morbidity and mortality rates than normal-weight but sedentary individuals.[12]

As aerobic exercise improves the fitness of the cardio-respiratory system, it helps protect against diseases of the heart, lungs and blood vessels that constitute the biggest killers in developed countries. This is why engaging in regular aerobic exercise is so important.

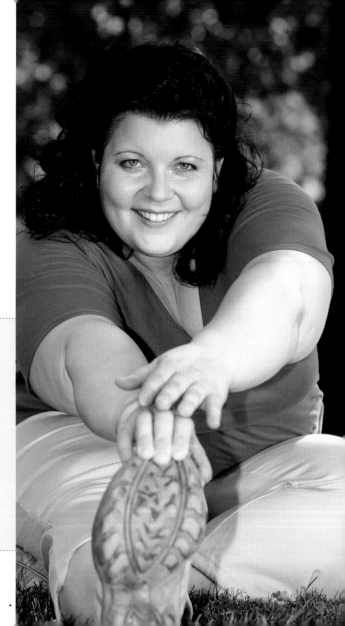

› More is better

While the current guidelines for most developed countries recommend 30 minutes of moderate-intensity aerobic exercise per day, growing evidence urges that more is better. Without wanting to be discouraging or overwhelming, especially given that in the United States only about one in four adults achieve the current guidelines, several studies now indicate that "30 minutes a day" may not be enough. [13]

If this amount of activity seems excessive, it is only because we have become so accustomed to sedentary living. We have come to think of sitting around and not moving as "normal" but this is not the way our bodies see it. We are made to move!

The expert panel went on to suggest that formerly obese individuals who want to keep the weight off may need to perform in the order of 60 to 90 minutes of moderate-intensity physical activity every day! This recommendation is in line with the findings of the National Weight Control Registry, which aimed to study the success secrets of individuals who lose weight and keep it off. The Registry now includes more than 5000 members who have lost an average of 73 pounds (33 kilograms) and maintained the loss for more than five years. One of the common practices of these success stories is that they engage in about one hour of physical activity every day. Other secrets of success reported by the members include eating a low-energy diet, eating breakfast regularly, self-monitoring weight, and maintaining a consistent eating pattern across weekdays and weekends. [14]

So 30 minutes of moderate-intensity aerobic exercise per day, which can be broken down into 10-minute chunks, is a tremendously beneficial pursuit. But—if you are able—more is better.

An expert panel review has suggested that 45 to 60 minutes of moderate-intensity activity is probably required to prevent people living in developed countries becoming overweight or obese.

STEP 3: Toughen up

There are many misconceptions associated with strength-building exercises.

Most people think it is necessary to join a gym and lift heavy weights. But strength-building exercises can be performed effectively using only your own body weight or simple aids that can be found around your home, such as cans of food or water bottles.

A second misconception about strength-building exercises is that they are only for young males. In reality, it is probably the opposite demographic—older females—who stand to benefit most from engaging in regular muscle-strengthening exercises. But whatever your age or gender, these exercises offer significant benefits:

> **Muscle-strengthening exercises tone the muscles and excite the nerves.**

It is good to have strong, toned muscles. Regularly performing strength-building exercises can greatly increase strength, which in turn can improve functionality. This can be especially important for elderly people, who discover that having the strength to get out of their chair unaided or retrieve items from high cupboards greatly improves their quality of life. Simple abilities make a big difference.

As we age, we tend to experience a loss of muscle tissue—an undesirable condition known as sarcopenia. However, strength-building exercises effectively counter this process.

Regularly performing strength-building exercises can greatly increase strength, which in turn can improve functionality.

A common fear among females that strength-building exercises will make them "big and bulky" is unfounded. Young males who want to experience this effect have to work extremely hard to achieve it and they have vastly greater concentrations of muscle-building testosterone in their system. If completed as recommended, strength-building exercise will improve muscle tone and increase strength without causing the muscles to "bulk up."

Improvements in strength occur quickly when someone engages in strength-building exercises for the first time, largely due to positive changes

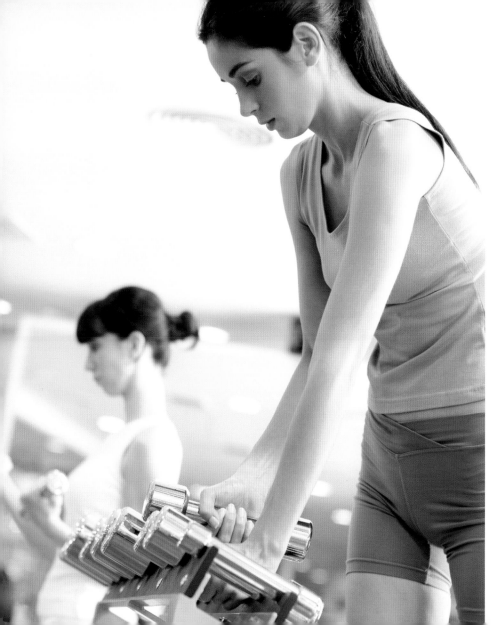

in the nervous system. Strength-building exercises are therefore not only good for our muscles, they also make our nerves "come alive"–and not just in the nerves leading to the muscles in our limbs. There is evidence that strength-building exercises aid brain health and can prevent cognitive decline.[15]

> **Muscle-strengthening exercises increase bone strength.**

It is not only muscles that grow stronger in response to strength-building exercises. All of the structures that support the muscles also toughen up, including the bones to which the muscles are attached.[16]

Bone strength becomes a major concern as we age because our bones begin to decrease in density after our third decade of life–and this speeds up even more in women after menopause.[17] Weak bones are obviously more susceptible to fracturing, which is a real problem especially among the elderly as our sense of balance gets worse as we age, making us more prone to falling. About one-third of adults over the age of 65 fall at least once per year and many of these falls result in

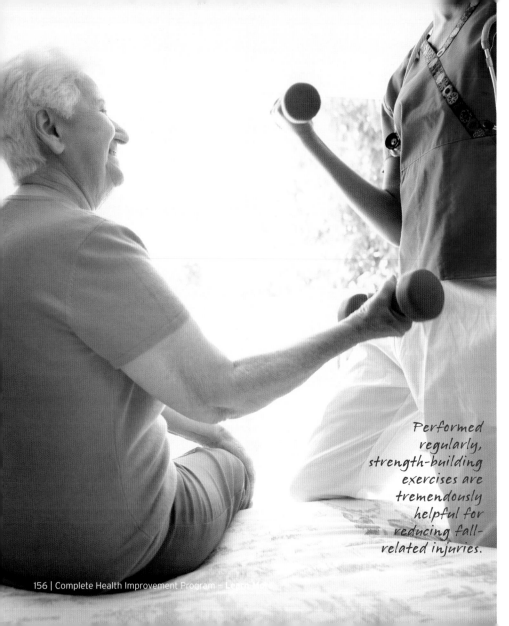

Performed regularly, strength-building exercises are tremendously helpful for reducing fall-related injuries.

fractures—about 90 per cent of hip fractures are fall-related.[18]

Performed regularly, strength-building exercises are tremendously helpful for reducing fall-related injuries. First, increased muscular strength and control achieved through regular strength training makes falling less likely. Second, by increasing bone density and strength, there is a reduced likelihood of a fracture even if a fall does occur.

> **Muscle-strengthening exercises can increase your metabolism.**

Toned muscles burn more energy, so strength-building exercises can increase your metabolic rate. This is extremely important for weight management as your resting metabolic rate—the speed at which your body burns energy when you are relaxed and doing nothing—contributes as much as 70 per cent of your daily energy expenditure.[19] Increasing your metabolic rate by just a few per cent can result in the body burning a lot more energy throughout the day—and night! If you burn energy at a faster rate, you are less likely to be overweight. For this reason, strength-building exercises are recommended as part of an effective weight-loss and maintenance program.

STEP 4: Stretch it out

The final ingredient of the optimal active lifestyle involves exercises designed to promote flexibility. The great thing about stretching exercises is they are simple to perform, can be executed almost anywhere and, best of all, require little effort or time.

Suppleness becomes increasingly important as we age because our body tissue has a tendency to stiffen, causing muscle tension, imbalance and pain. Performing regular stretching exercises can assist in maintaining good flexibility.

It is commonly believed that the best time to stretch is before exercise but there is no evidence that stretching before exercise decreases the chance of injury. It may even reduce the amount of force your muscles can produce if you are doing high-intensity exercise.[20]

It is probably better to stretch after you have exercised and are warmed up—or just any time you have a few spare minutes in the day. Stretches don't take long and you can do them almost anywhere. Regular stretching will not only make you more supple but can also help with muscle relaxation and reduce muscle soreness. There is some evidence that stretching actually produces an analgesic (pain-relieving) effect.[21]

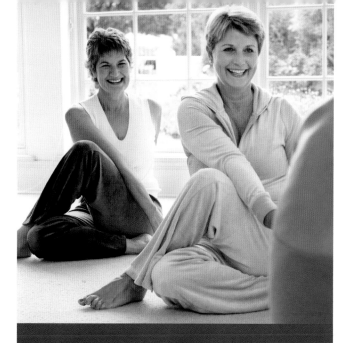

MAKE THE STRETCH

There are various forms of stretching but the safest and easiest is referred to as "static" stretching. A static stretch is one in which the muscle is taken to the end of its range of motion—it should not be painful—and held in that position for 10 to 30 seconds. The stretch is then repeated three or four times.

For best results, aim to perform a series of stretching exercises that target different parts of the body two or more times each week.

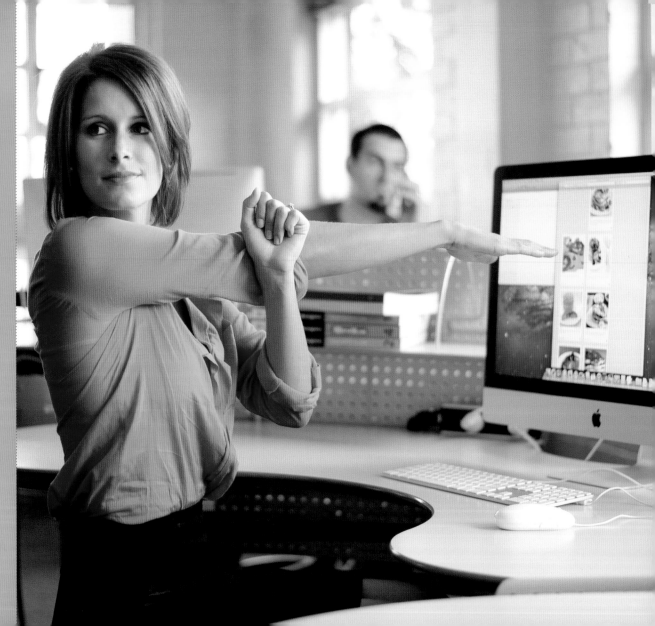

KEY POINTS

To avoid the perils of inactivity and enjoy the pleasures of the optimal active life-style, be intentional about:

› Breaking up prolonged sit time.

› Engaging in regular aerobic activities—at least 30 minutes of moderate-intensity physical activity a day.

› Performing exercises that develop muscular strength and improve flexibility twice per week.

Chapter Eleven References

1   Patel, A, et al (2010), "Leisure Time Spent Sitting in Relation to Total Mortality in a Prospective Cohort of US Adults," *American Journal of Epidemiology*, Vol 172, pages 419–29.

2   Adapted from National Heart Foundation of Australia (2011), "Sitting less for adults," <www.heartfoundation.org.au/SiteCollectionDocuments/HW-PA-SittingLess-Adults.pdf>.

3   Stamatakis, E, et al (2011), "Screen-Based Entertainment Time, All-Cause Mortality, and Cardiovascular Events: Population-Based Study With Ongoing Mortality and Hospital Events Follow-Up," *Journal of the American College of Cardiology*, Vol 57, pages 292–9.

4   Hamilton, M, et al (2008), "Too Little Exercise and Too Much Sitting: Inactivity Physiology and the Need for New Recommendations on Sedentary Behavior," *Current Cardiovascular Risk Reports*, Vol 2, pages 292–8.

5   Healy, G N, et al (2008), "Breaks in sedentary time—beneficial associations with metabolic risk," *Diabetes Care*, Vol 31, No 4, pages 661–6.

6   National Heart Foundation of Australia (2011), "Sitting less for adults," <www.heartfoundation.org.au/SiteCollectionDocuments/HW-PA-SittingLess-Adults.pdf>.

7   United States Department of Health and Human Services, "2008 Physical Activity Guidelines for Americans," <www.health.gov/paguidelines>.

8   Norton, K, et al (2010), "Position statement on physical activity and exercise intensity terminology," *Journal of Science and Medicine in Sport*, Vol 13, pages 496–502.

9   ibid.

10 Fletcher, G F, et al (1996), "Statement on Exercise: Benefits and Recommendations for Physical Activity Programs for All Americans," *Circulation*, Vol 94, pages 857–62.

11 Lee, D C, et al (2009), "Does physical activity ameliorate the health hazards of obesity?" British Journal of Sports Medicine, Vol 43, pages 49–51; Lee, D C, et al (2011), "Long-Term Effects of Changes in Cardiorespiratory Fitness and Body Mass Index on All-Cause and Cardiovascular Disease Mortality in Men: The Aerobics Center Longitudinal Study," *Circulation*, Vol 124, pages 2483–90.

12 Blair, S N, and S Brodney (1999), "Effects of physical inactivity and obesity on morbidity and mortality: current evidence and research issues," *Medicine and Science in Sports and Exercise*, Vol 31 No 11 Supplement, pages S646–62. 1999.

13 Saris, et al (2003), "How much physical activity is enough to prevent unhealthy weight gain? Outcome of the IASO 1st Stock Conference and consensus statement," *Obesity Reviews*, Vol 4, pages 101–14.

14 National Weight Control Registry <www.nwcr.ws>

15 Liu-Ambrose, T, and M G Donaldson (2009), "Exercise and cognition in older adults: is there a role for resistance training programmes?" *British Journal of Sports Medicine*, Vol 43, pages 25–7.

16 Nybo, L, et al (2010), "High-Intensity Training versus Traditional Exercise Interventions for Promoting Health," *Medicine and Science in Sports and Exercise*, Vol 42, No 10, pages 1951–8.

17 Carter, N D, et al (2001), "Exercise in the Prevention of Falls in Older People. A Systematic Literature Review Examining the Rationale and the Evidence," *Sports Medicine*, Vol 31, No 6, pages 427–38.

18 ibid.

19 Stiegler, P, and A Cunliffe (2006), "The Role of Diet and Exercise for the Maintenance of Fat-Free Mass and Resting Metabolic Rate During Weight Loss," *Sports Medicine*, Vol 36 No 3, pages 239–62.

20 Shrier, I (2004), "Does Stretching Improve Performance? A Systematic and Critical Review of the Literature," *Clinical Journal of Sport Medicine*, Vol 14 No 5, pages 267–73.

21 Shrier, I (2007), "Does stretching help prevent injuries?" in D MacAuley and T M Best (eds), *Evidence-based Sports Medicine (2nd Edition)*, Blackwell Publishing, Massachusetts.

Get Set for Success

You have begun a journey toward living more and your efforts are to be applauded. However, the real challenge of adopting healthier behaviors is sustaining them. All too often as we progress on a journey of behavior change, we run into roadblocks that can arrest our progress and even derail us. In this section, we consider some of the common roadblocks individuals encounter and strategies for negotiating them.

Chapter Twelve starts by asking, "Why we do what we do?" and shows that our beliefs can radically shape our behaviors, highlighting the importance of reframing our beliefs to serve, rather than hinder, us in our quest to live more. This chapter also considers the value and motivational properties of goal setting.

Chapter Thirteen looks at how unforgiveness can contribute to poor health, while practising forgiveness can be healing. This chapter considers what forgiveness is really about and how we need to forgive—both others and ourselves—to truly live.

Chapter Fourteen demonstrates that our genes are not our fate and that our past doesn't need to equal our future by highlighting exciting discoveries from the field of epigenetics.

Chapter Fifteen creates an awareness of how our environment—political, economic, social and physical—has a tremendous influence on our lifestyle habits, and how we can take steps to create an environment that supports us on our journey to living healthier and better.

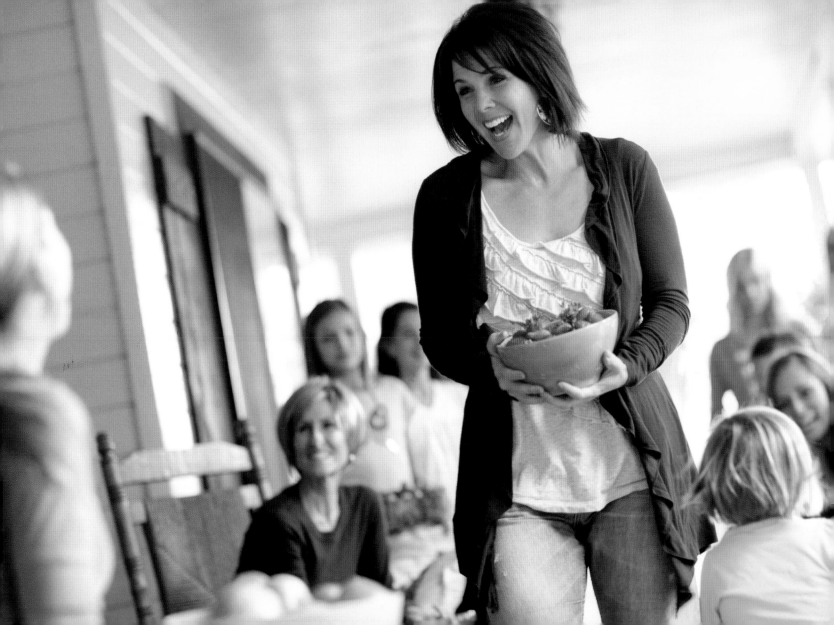

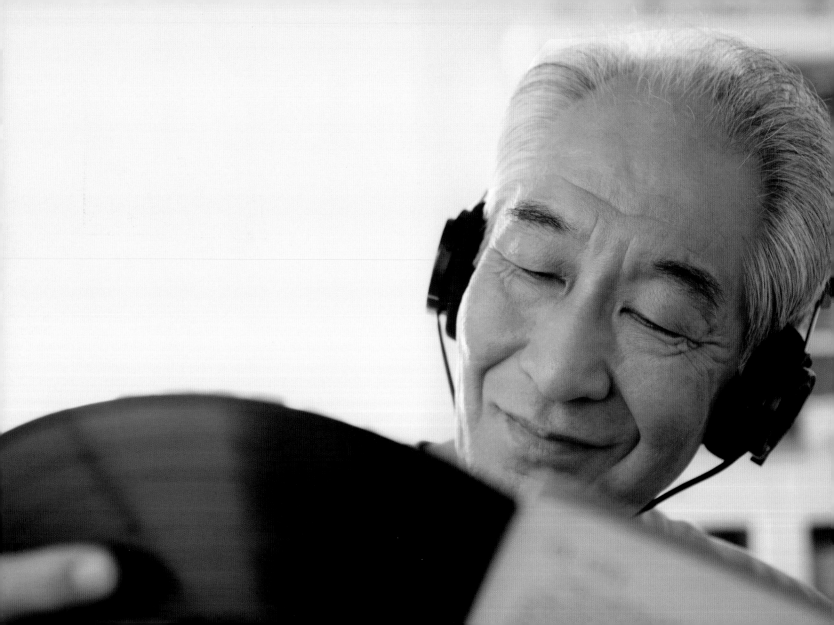

Chapter Twelve

Become What You Believe

Thousands of years ago, Aristotle came up with the idea that we humans are primarily motivated by pleasure and pain—we do things to achieve pleasure and we do things to avoid pain. It is all about the carrot and the stick! While there are many theories about why humans do what they do and how we can change it,[1] this simplistic view gives us a good place to start our exploration of what drives our behaviors.

To state it simply, we do what we do for a feeling—and there is good reason for this. Neurophysiologists, who study how the brain is put together and works, have discovered that the part of our brain responsible for our emotions (or feelings), referred to as the limbic system, is also primarily responsible for our drives and behaviors.[2] This explains why a strong feeling toward something excites our best efforts, whereas when we have no feelings toward a particular thing we are not inspired to action.

For example, consider what people will do when gripped by the strong feelings of love or fear. People don't have any difficulty motivating themselves to do whatever it takes to secure the source of their love or escape the source of their fear. On the other hand, when we lack feelings we are apathetic and unmotivated. Ask a couch potato why they don't get exercise and they will tell you quite frankly that they don't *feel* like it!

As a side note, it is an interesting fact that the limbic system—our emotional brain—is highly stimulated by smell and taste.[3] This explains in part why people "comfort eat." Essentially

> *People don't have any difficultly motivating themselves to do whatever it takes to secure the source of their love or escape the source of their fear.*

when our limbic system gets emotionally down or stressed and wants a pick-me-up, it drives us to eat. Unfortunately, it tends to drive us to eat sweet and fatty foods that are not helpful when it comes to optimizing our health! As Dr Neal Barnard points out, no-one says, "I feel so upset that I just need to eat a whole head of broccoli!"[4] Once again, this highlights the fact that we do what we do for a feeling.

Learn to love it!

That feelings powerfully drive our behavior is an important consideration when it comes to being motivated long-term, and hence experiencing long-term behavior change. To successfully adopt a new behavior, we need to come to a point where the new behavior is pleasurable. If it is unpleasant—especially if it is painful—it will almost be impossible to sustain over time. The behavior-change experts who wrote *Change Anything* say that the first step toward experiencing long-term success is to learn to love the new behavior.[5]

Learning to find pleasure in a new behavior can take time and one reason many people fail is because they don't persist long enough. Consider exercise as an example. Many people associate exercise with *pain*. Is it any wonder so many people are completely unmotivated to do it? Unfortunately, when an individual first starts to become more active, it may not be entirely pleasant—especially since many people push themselves too hard, too early. As a result, they confirm their belief that exercise is something to be endured, not enjoyed.

So, when becoming more active, it is important we do whatever we can to make the experience as less burdensome as possible. If you are not a morning person, don't exercise in the morning! If you are a social person, don't do it alone if you can help it. And keep reminding yourself that you only need to engage in moderate-intensity activity to reap great rewards! In time, our brain and body adjust, and we come to find the experience pleasurable. Exercise has even been shown to boost our endorphin levels, which can have mood enhancing effects. At this point, being active becomes sustainable.

In time, our brain and body adjust, and we come to find the experience pleasurable. At this point, being active becomes sustainable.

The same principle applies to transitioning to healthier eating patterns. In the early stages of change, we might find our new food choices less pleasurable than our former unhealthy choices. For this reason, it is so important to learn tasty recipes to make your new food choices as pleasurable as possible. It is not sustainable to go through life eating foods that are unpalatable to you!

Interestingly, in time your taste buds change and you will begin to experience the joy of new and subtle flavors, while the foods you once found pleasure in no longer hold their appeal. For example, after eating salt-reduced foods for a relatively short period of time, your palate will find the salty foods you once loved much too salty. Similarly, an eating plan full of healthy, wholesome foods with their fresh flavors can also leave you feeling deeply nourished. At this point, the new behaviors become entirely sustainable.

To help secure long-term success in your journey toward optimal health, discover ways of making the new healthy behaviors as pleasurable as possible.

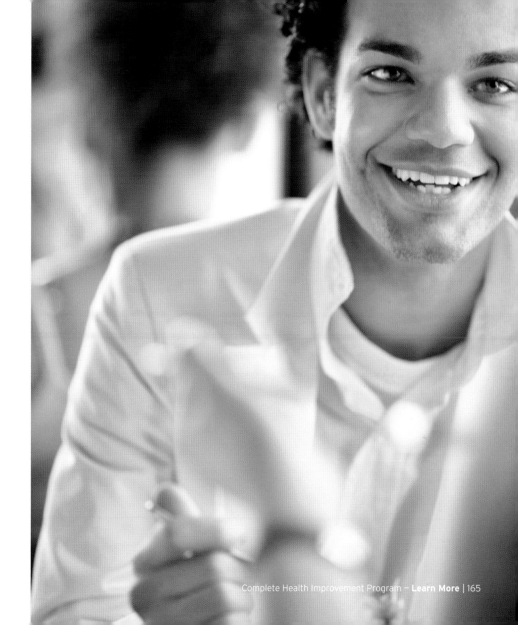

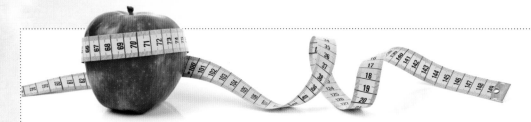

HOW TO KEEP IT LOST

The National Weight Control Registry is an initiative of researchers from Brown Medical School and the University of Colorado.[7] The researchers have been studying the secrets of successful weight loss by identifying individuals who have lost a significant portion of their body weight and kept it off for an extended period of time. The registry now includes information from more than 5000 individuals who have lost an average 73 pounds (about 33 kilograms) and have kept it off for longer than five years.

So what makes these success stories so successful? They tend to:

1. Eat foods of low energy density, including a hearty breakfast.

2. Weigh themselves regularly, indicating that self-monitoring is important.

3. Watch less than 10 hours of television per week.

4. Engage in about one hour of physical activity most days.

But these are strategies we all know! So why doesn't everyone carry out these behaviors? And what makes these individuals different?

It probably has something to do with beliefs about themselves that they have changed or reframed. Individuals who achieve permanent weight loss can be heard to say things like "This is just who I am now" and "I no longer look in the mirror and see an obese person." Such statements communicate a changed belief about themselves and who they are. This new belief serves as the new reference for how they feel and how they behave.

When they come to see themselves as a normal-weight individual, if they start gaining weight again it causes unpleasant feelings that drive behaviors until they return to where their new belief tells them they should be. In order to experience permanent change, we often need to change what we believe.

Become what you believe

As we have seen, our feelings drive our behaviors, so why do different people in similar circumstances feel differently, then behave differently? To illustrate, consider punctuality. Some individuals are sticklers for time; others are not. If a diligently time-conscious person is running late, they will be overcome with unpleasant feelings, becoming agitated, anxious and frustrated. As a result, they start behaving in ways that will get them to their destination as quickly as possible so they can be relieved of these feelings. They might walk or drive faster—even more recklessly. On the other hand, a tardy individual generally does not experience such unpleasant feelings when running late—certainly not enough to modify their behavior—so they feel no compulsion to hurry.

But why do some feel stressed, anxious and agitated when running late, while others do not?

At the heart of it, time-aware individuals have certain beliefs about being late, like "It is rude to be late" or "Being late shows you don't care" or "Being late is a poor reflection on you as a person." Those beliefs cause the unpleasant feelings, which in turn drive their hurried behaviors. By contrast, an individual who does not hold such beliefs is not overcome with unpleasant feelings when running late and does not feel compelled to hurry. Perhaps an individual with a belief such as "It is polite to get there a little late in order to give the other person more time to get ready" will actually experience pleasant feelings when running late, so are even more inclined to never be on time! Our beliefs serve as the reference for how we feel, then those feelings drive our behaviors. Or to state it simply, *beliefs drive behavior.*[6]

Whether we realize it or not, we have many beliefs that serve as reference points for how we feel in certain situations, which in turn cause us to behave in certain ways. We might never have consciously thought about many of the beliefs we hold but they can have a powerful influence over our life, perhaps even acting as roadblocks to our journey toward optimal living.

Consider the example of weight loss. Many people lose weight, only to regain it in following months and years. While physiological

Our beliefs serve as the reference for how we feel, then those feelings drive our behaviors.

explanations have been proposed, psychology plays a huge part. For example, when someone loses a significant amount of body weight but does not change their belief about who they are, they tend to gain it back.

The psychology behind this is fascinating. As they start gaining the weight back, it doesn't result in unpleasant feelings—they don't believe they are that thinner person anyway!—so they are unlikely to change their behaviors to keep the weight off. But for some individuals, being thinner than what they believe they should be—how they see themselves— can actually cause underlying unpleasant feelings that will compel them to behave in ways that will sabotage their weight-loss success, until they get back to where they believe they should be. Our beliefs can act like a thermostat setting we keep returning to.

So where do we get these beliefs about ourselves that so powerfully shape our lives? They are instilled in us by two influential teachers:

Credible sources are individuals we find believable as we journey through life, starting predominately with our parents and guardians, then including our teachers, peers and significant others who may or may not be related or close to us.

It is important to distinguish between "credible" and "incredible" sources. For example, watching Olympic athletes perform is inspiring, but it is unlikely to change what we believe we are capable of—after all, they are "incredible." For a source to be "credible" they have to be "like us" in some significant way. For this reason, a dietitian who counsels on weight loss is more credible and likely to make an individual believe they can do it if the dietitian themself has struggled with their own weight but has been successful.

Personal experiences also form our beliefs. Unfortunately, negative experiences are often more potent than positive ones—you tend to remember the time the dog bit you more vividly than the times you patted it happily.

The key to changing and reframing beliefs is found in these same processes, utilizing positive influences by actively seeking out credible sources and positive experiences that can help us forge beliefs about the true worth of ourselves that will serve us well in life. It can take time and effort to change beliefs about ourselves, but it is important that we do to achieve long-term success.

You are worth it

In the context of the optimal lifestyle, three beliefs are fundamentally important in order to experience long-term success:

1. It is important that I prioritize my health and wellbeing.

We will be unmotivated to take positive steps unless we believe it is important that we do.[8] Unfortunately, many people have to come to a point of pain before they embrace this belief and are motivated to take action. The good news is it is never too late to benefit from the optimal lifestyle.

2. This will work for me.

Unless you believe change is possible and that you are capable of achieving it, you will clearly have no inclination to strive for it.[9] This belief in your ability to make changes and improve your health is referred to as health-related self-efficacy. Individuals with a high level of self-efficacy are more inclined to initiate better lifestyle choices, persist for longer and are less likely to slip back to their old ways.[10] The Complete Health Improvement Program (CHIP) is designed to help you develop self-efficacy by connecting you with others, just like yourself—"credible" sources—who have experienced CHIP success. At the same time, CHIP aims to provide you with a first-hand positive experience of transforming your health.

3. I deserve CHIP success.

This third core belief required for long-term success often goes unrecognized. For many people, credible sources and unfortunate life experiences have taught them that they do not deserve good things in life. Tragically, they have formed a belief that they are not valuable and of importance. Individuals who have developed such a belief have no ambition to strive for a better life.

But every person has tremendous value and incredible worth, and deserves a life of health and wholeness. Worth is not based on what we do or what we own or how broken we may be. *You* are valuable just because you are, and *you* deserve health and wholeness. Embracing this belief will empower you to overcome many roadblocks in the way of living your best life.

Goals

Armed with a high level of health-related self-efficacy and a strong belief in your self-worth, you are still unlikely to experience vibrant health unless you have it as a goal—and have an action plan for achieving it. Setting goals can greatly enhance your likelihood of success because:

› Goals give you something to direct your attention to.

› Goals energize your level of engagement and commitment.

› Goals make you more persistent in the face of adversity.

› Goals give you a rewarding sense of satisfaction when you attain them.[11]

One helpful approach to setting goals is to apply the SMART goals principle.[12] SMART goals are:

Specific: Goals need to be specific if they are to offer us clear direction. Having a vague goal like "I want to improve my health" is not as motivating as "I want to lose 5 per cent of my body weight."

Measurable: Choosing a goal that has a measureable outcome is more likely to create a higher level of engagement with an action plan than something that can't be clearly measured. As with the examples above, "losing 5 per cent of my body weight" sets a clear target, whereas "improving my health" is more difficult to judge in the absence of some quantifiable measures. This is why CHIP includes measureable outcomes. While you might *feel* better, you can also see measurable evidence of the improvements.

Achievable: "I want to go to the Olympics!"—while this might be an achievable goal for some, it is too ambitious for most of us. Challenging goals can be great, but if they are unattainable we set ourselves up for failure and dissatisfaction, which is extremely demotivating. Choose goals that will stretch you, but not break you.

Relevant: The goals we set for ourselves need to be worthwhile and meaningful, as well as relevant to what we are trying to achieve. Setting yourself a goal at the beginning of CHIP of "renovating the bathroom" is not likely to help your CHIP journey. Goals need to be relevant to the task at hand, perhaps "renovating my health."

Timely: One of the greatest causes of procrastination is the "one day" mentality: "I will get fitter—*one day*" or "*One day* I will start eating better." For goals to be most helpful, they need to be time-framed to create a sense of urgency and help structure a plan to achieve them. It is good to set both short-term and long-term goals that give us something to aim for daily and, perhaps, yearly. Short-term goals can be stepping-stones to encourage us on our journey toward our long-term goals.

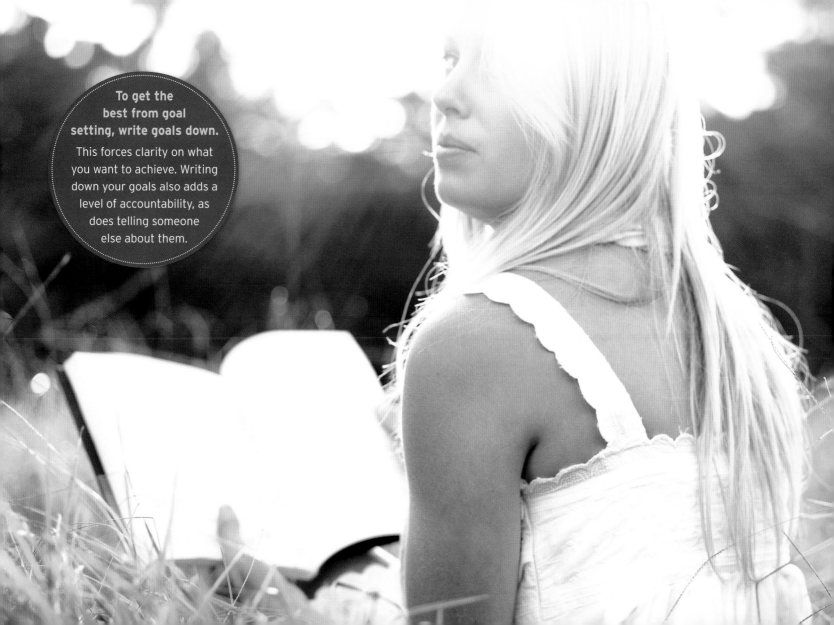

To get the best from goal setting, write goals down.

This forces clarity on what you want to achieve. Writing down your goals also adds a level of accountability, as does telling someone else about them.

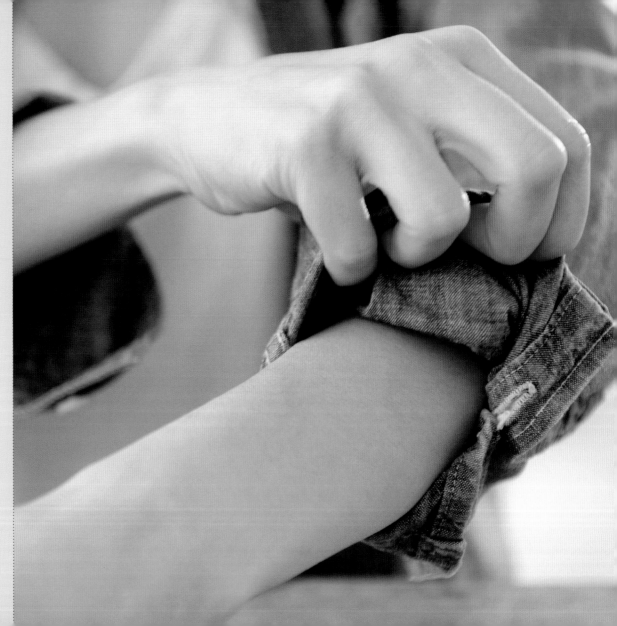

KEY POINTS

› Human behavior is often puzzling but we tend to be motivated by feelings– we do things to achieve pleasure and avoid pain.

› As our beliefs act as a reference for how we feel in certain situations, beliefs powerfully drive our behaviors. Accordingly, successfully adopting positive new behaviors often requires changing our beliefs about the importance of making the change, our ability to make the change and how deserving we are of the change.

› Setting SMART goals can be extremely helpful for nurturing a journey of positive behavior change.

Chapter Twelve References

1   Elder, J (1999), "Theories and Intervention Approaches to Health-Behavior Change in Primary Care," *American Journal of Preventative Medicine,* Vol 17 No 4, pages 275–84.

2   Clark, D L, et al (2010), *The Brain and Behavior: An Introduction to Behavioral Neuroanatomy,* Cambridge University Press.

3   ibid.

4   Barnard, N (2003), *Breaking the Food Seduction: The Hidden Reasons Behind Food Cravings–And 7 Steps to End Them Naturally,* St Martins Griffin.

5   Patterson, K, et al (2011), *Change Anything: The New Science of Personal Success,* Piatkus.

6   Hale, E D, et al (2007), "The Common-Sense Model of self-regulation of health and illness: how can we use it to understand and respond to our patients' needs?" *Rheumatology,* Vol 46 No 6, pages 904–6.

7   Wing, R, and S Phelan (2005), "Long-term weight loss maintenance," *American Journal of Clinical Nutrition,* Vol 82 No 1, pages 222S-225S; see also <www.nwcr.ws>.

8   Janz, N K, and M H Becker (1984), "The health belief model: a decade later," *Health Education Quarterly,* Vol 11 No 1, pages 1–47.

9   ibid.

10   Schwarzer, R (2008), "Modeling Health Behavior Change: How to Predict and Modify the Adoption and Maintenance of Health Behaviors," *Applied Psychology,* Vol 57 No 1, pages 1–29.

11   Locke, E, and G Latham (2002), "Building a Practically Useful Theory of Goal Setting and Task Motivation: A 35-Year Odyssey," *American Psychologist,* Vol 57 No 9, pages 705–17.

12   Doran, G (1981), "There's a S.M.A.R.T. way to write management's goals and objectives," *Management Review,* Vol 70 No 11, pages 35–6; Meyer, P (2003), "What would you do if you knew you couldn't fail? Creating S.M.A.R.T. Goals," *Attitude Is Everything: If You Want to Succeed Above and Beyond,* Meyer Resource Group, Incorporated.

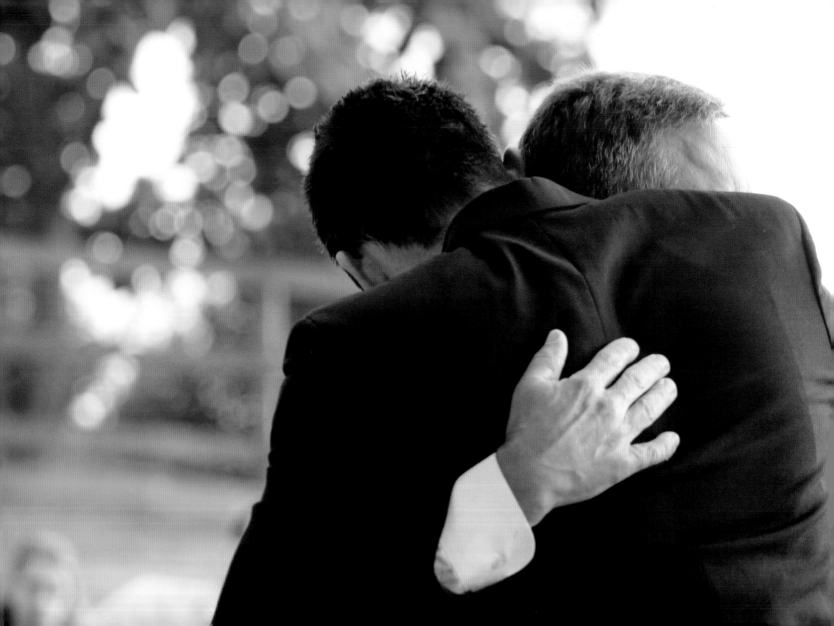

Chapter Thirteen

Practising Forgiveness

The interaction between mind and body is fascinating. The impact our thoughts, feelings and emotions have on our physiology and physical health demands the attention of anyone interested in optimal wellbeing. Research has shown that a healthy outlook tends to result in greater physical health, while an unhealthy outlook is linked to chronic illness and premature death.[1] One way this works is that our emotional states result in the release of a variety of hormones into our blood stream—affecting the function and wellbeing of crucial organs throughout our body.

Anger, bitterness and resentment are emotions that have attracted the attention of researchers in recent years. So powerful are their effects on the human body, they are emotions with the potential to kill. It seems we hear more and more news stories of angry, aggressive people killing total strangers who have inadvertently upset them in some minor way in traffic. But even if you are not the violent type, the grudge you might be bitterly holding onto still has the potential to kill—and you are the potential victim. At the least, it's diminishing your wellbeing and holding you back from living a full and abundant life.

Even if you are not the violent type, the grudge you might be bitterly holding onto still has the potential to kill—and you are the potential victim.

Anger and your body

When you get angry, your body's "fight-or-flight" response is activated, as it is when you experience fear, excitement or anxiety. Your adrenal glands produce a deluge of hormones—particularly, adrenaline and cortisol—that course through your body. Blood flow is concentrated in the muscles, ready for physical exertion—whether flight or fight. Your heart rate, blood pressure, respiration, body temperature and perspiration all increase,[2] as do the levels of glucose and fat in your blood stream.[3] Your body is ready for action—ready to respond to the problem at hand.

› Real or imagined—it doesn't matter

Have you ever woken from a frightening dream with your heart nearly pounding right out of your chest? The dream wasn't real, but your brain believed it was.

Similarly, when it comes to the impact of anger on your body, truth is irrelevant. Your body does not care if you are actually experiencing an infuriating event right here and now, or if you are just thinking about one that once happened. It still tells your body to get ready for action and you will still experience the physical effects of the emotions your thoughts produce.

› Long-term anger

Getting angry is not necessarily a problem—but staying angry is. Our bodies are well designed to handle a stressful event that is quickly resolved. But researchers have found that prolonged anger has a devastating effect on physical health. Anger that does not go away can physically damage us because our body has insufficient recovery time, if any. Health problems that have been linked to unresolved anger include insomnia, depression, high blood pressure, heart attack and stroke.[4]

The body's response to anger—increased blood

pressure, heart rate, and glucose and fat in the blood stream—wears away at the heart and cardiovascular system, and may damage the artery walls.[5] People who are angry or hostile have elevated levels of catecholamines (including cortisol), which result in faster development of fatty deposits in the heart and carotid arteries,[6] and are known to produce coronary spasm and arrhythmias.[7]

It seems clear: being an angry person is bad for your physical health, and managing anger can improve your physical health.

The findings on anger

In recent years, the health effects of anger have been the focus of increasing research:

> Following a decades-long study, researchers from Johns Hopkins University School of Medicine reported that young men who react quickly to stress with anger had three times the normal risk of developing early heart disease, and were five times as likely to have early heart attacks.[8]

> A 2007 study found that high levels of anger increased men's risk of developing high blood pressure—a well-accepted risk factor for coronary heart disease.[9]

> After reviewing data from 44 scientific studies, researchers concluded that anger and hostility resulted in healthy people being more likely to develop coronary heart disease (CHD). They also concluded that anger and hostility led to poor outcomes for people who already had CHD. They believed that managing anger and hostility would be useful for both the prevention and treatment of CHD.[10]

Two options for dealing with anger:

Option 1: Stay angry

Almost all the unhealthy emotions we experience stem from damaged relationships, the casualty of some upsetting event. Hurt and resentment—steps on the anger continuum—are feelings we seem to cling to. In fact, we experience negative emotions four to 10 times more intensely than we experience positive ones.

We seem to relish going over the upsetting event again and again in our thoughts. We might fantasize about what we wish we had said or what we might say at some future opportunity to even the score. But each time we do, we re-live the emotions that our brain believes require an urgent response. While we wait in vain for the other party's admission of guilt or request for forgiveness, we keep ourselves angry and bitter, placing immense pressure on our mental and physical health: "Unforgiveness is like carrying around a red-hot rock with the intention of throwing it at the person who caused you the hurt. But as you wait . . . the sizzling rock burns and scars your hand. Wouldn't it be wiser just to let the rock fall to the ground? Forgiveness is the skill of letting go."[11]

Option 2: Release yourself from anger

When you remain angry with a person, feeling hurt and bitter, you are essentially handcuffing yourself to the one you blame. You are locking yourself in your own personal prison of unhappiness, while the other person might be oblivious to your festering resentment. Another way of thinking about it: you simply cannot take a poison pill and hope the other person dies. The question is: do you want your life controlled by some other person or event that took place in the distant past? Or do you want your life to be in your control? Only you can set yourself free.

The unpopular alternative to holding on to grudges, resentment and anger is to forgive! In the context of living a healthy life, the word *forgiveness* refers to our ability to let go of painful experiences from our past, to move on and put them behind us instead of dragging them around everywhere we go. This is known as "personal forgiveness" and research has shown that practising personal forgiveness reduces anger and can reverse some diseases, including high blood pressure.[12]

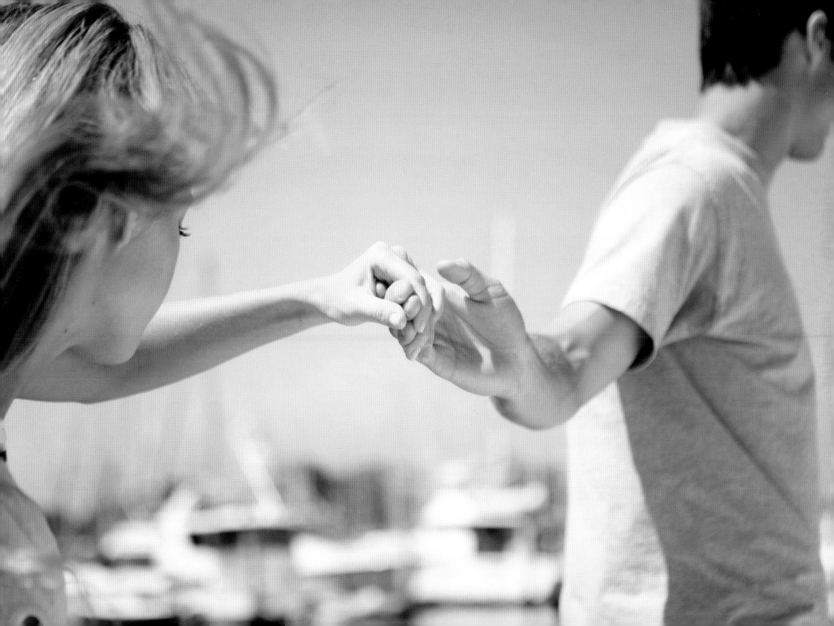

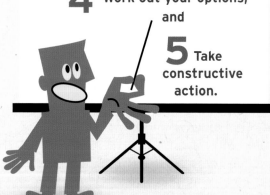

Five steps to handle anger

Counsellor and author Gary Chapman suggests a five-step process when anger rears its head:[13]

1 Acknowledge your anger;

2 Restrain your immediate response;

3 Identify what you're actually angry about;

4 Work out your options; and

5 Take constructive action.

What forgiveness isn't

Forgiveness is an unpopular option because people don't want to let the offender "get away with" the "wrong" they have done. They fear that by forgiving, they will somehow diminish the other person's guilt. But forgiveness does not make a wrong act right, nor condone or excuse the wrong act. It does not automatically return trust to a relationship–this must still be earned. Personal forgiveness is simply about freeing yourself, because you're worth it. It recognizes that by holding on to your resentment, you are making *your* life a misery, not theirs.

Of course, when an offence first occurs, our options include more than "be angry" or "let it go." Ideally, the conflict should be resolved.

As you consider your options, sometimes you'll decide that resolving the problem isn't one of them. That's when you choose to either stew in your own anger or learn to let it go and move on.

The process of personal forgiveness

Personal forgiveness is a process that takes time and usually needs to be cycled through a number of times for any given painful situation.

› Choices

Life is more about choices than circumstances. What we make of our circumstances is determined by the choices we make. And the more we select a certain choice, the easier it becomes as it is increasingly hard-wired in our brain. This is true of both healthy and unhealthy choices.

Also, consider unconscious versus conscious choices. We can respond reactively (unconsciously) to a painful event, or we can pause and make a conscious choice about how to respond. We have the freedom and power to choose our responses to the circumstances life throws at us. We can angrily blame another for our unhappiness or we can take responsibility for moving forward with our lives.

› The "forgive-and-forget" myth

Forgetting a painful event is something that can rarely be achieved. The goal of personal forgiveness is to remember the painful event in a different way. It isn't about if you remember, but *how* you remember. Usually, the "grievance story" we have crafted through frequent re-telling is riddled with distortions, biases and incomplete details. Memories are often inaccurate. Two eyewitnesses can give significantly different testimonies. Two children from the same family remember vastly different childhoods. We should not be surprised that we may have a flawed recollection of what happened in a painful event.

› Reframing

Instead of forgetting what happened, we need to remember it in a different way. We need to reframe the event. This involves choosing what facts to include—and generally means enlarging our focus. Most people focus on facts that reinforce their existing point of view and ignore facts that challenge it.

Reframing requires us to focus on the facts from both perspectives. It is helpful to develop at least some understanding of the offender's circumstances at the time of the painful event. And it helps to recognize our own offences. If we realize that we can inadvertently do painful things, we can be more tolerant to others' failings.

Revising our story so it is more accurate is still only the beginning. Forgiveness—moving on—takes time and often requires cycling through this process several times. In the meantime, move toward your life goals.

Enjoy having the weight lifted from your shoulders and live the life you want to live!

It is helpful to develop at least some understanding of the offender's circumstances at the time of the painful event.

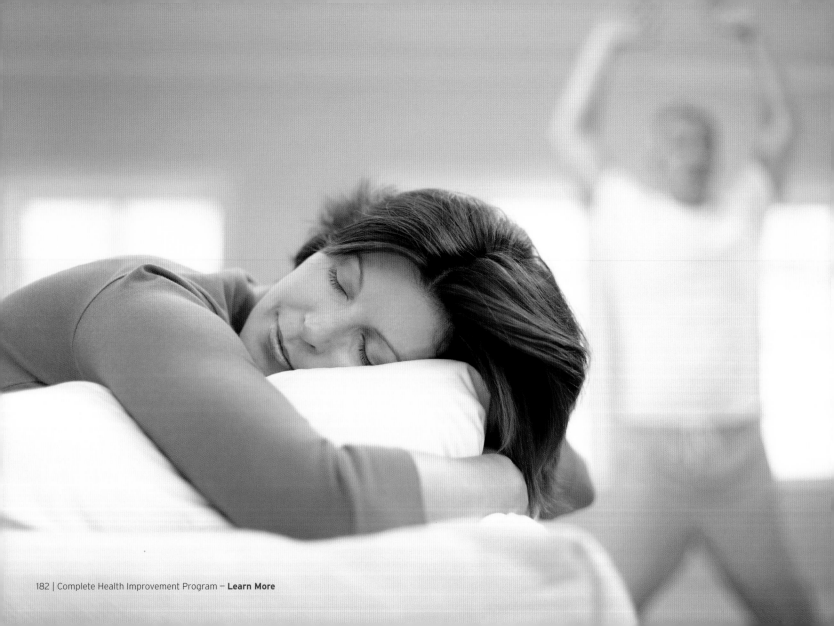

Forgiving yourself

Sometimes the hardest person to forgive is you. This can be especially true when we have begun making positive changes to our life and health, only to suddenly find ourselves back where we started.

Perhaps you single-handedly ate an entire packet of chocolate cookies. Before you start beating yourself up, remember that everybody makes mistakes. It is normal to suffer relapse.

Most people making changes in their lives progress through various "stages of change" in their journey.[14]

STAGES OF CHANGE *(relapse–can occur at any stage)*				
Pre-contemplation	**Contemplation**	**Preparation**	**Action**	**Maintenance/ Relapse**
Do you remember a time when you weren't concerned about your health or didn't see any need to change anything?	At some point, you began to consider the possibility that you needed to do something. Some people think about it for months, years or even their entire lives without progressing.	You began to prepare for the change—bought a pair of running shoes, researched gym memberships or began looking for healthy recipes.	Then you took action: perhaps you started walking during your lunch break. It was great! You felt good about yourself. You could feel your body toning up. You didn't get so puffed going up the hill.	But for how long were you able to maintain it? Were you derailed by a week of non-stop rain? The end-of-financial-year pressures in the office? A family crisis?

When people don't maintain their new health habit, they often feel like a failure. But the good news is that almost everyone struggles with maintenance! It's completely normal to be challenged by the obstacles of everyday life.

If you suffer a relapse, forgive yourself. Most people get derailed and everyone makes mistakes. A mistake is not a failure—it's a mistake. You can't change what has happened. Beating yourself up about it will not undo what has been done. Acknowledge that it's happened, learn from it what you can, then put it behind you and move forward, with a renewed commitment to your goal.

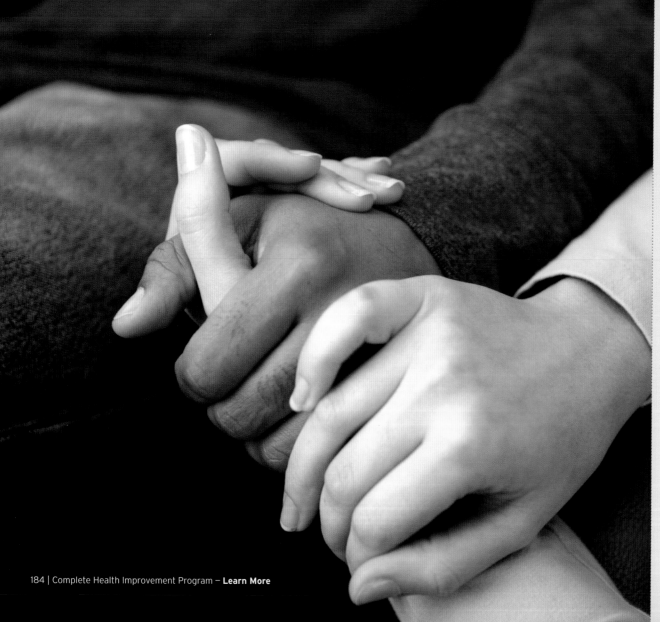

KEY POINTS

› No-one can avoid hurt. It's how we deal with it that matters: we can complain and blame, or forgive and live.

› Scientific and medical research is increasingly demonstrating the physical and health benefits of practising forgiveness.

› We also need to learn to forgive ourselves, particularly when seeking to make changes in our lives.

Chapter Thirteen References

1   Many of the ideas in this chapter are drawn, with permission, from Tibbits, D (2006), *Forgive to Live: How Forgiveness Can Save Your Life,* Thomas Nelson.

2   Better Health Channel (2012), "Anger—How it affects people," <www.betterhealth.vic.gov.au/bhcv2/bhcarticles.nsf/pages/Anger_how_it_affects_people>.

3   WebMD (2012), "How Anger Hurts Your Heart," <www.webmd.com/balance/stress-management/features/how-anger-hurts-your-heart>.

4   Better Health Channel, op cit.

5   WebMD, op cit.

6   Cleveland Clinic (2012), "Anger and Heart Attack," <http://my.clevelandclinic.org/heart/prevention/stress/anger.aspx>.

7   Adameova, A, et al (2009), "Role of the excessive amounts of circulating catecholamines and glucocorticoids in stress-induced heart disease," *Canadian Journal of Physiology and Pharmacology,* Vol 87 No 7, pages 493-514.

8   Chang, P, et al (2002), "Anger in Young Men and Subsequent Premature Cardiovascular Disease: The Precursors Study," *Archives of Internal Medicine,* Vol 162 No 8, pages 901-6.

9   Player, M S, et al (2007), "Psychosocial factors and progression from pre-hypertension to hypertension or coronary heart disease," *Annals of Family Medicine,* Vol 5 No 5, pages 403-11.

10 Chida, Y, and A Steptoe (2009), "The Association of Anger and Hostility with Future Coronary Heart Disease: A meta-analytic review of prospective evidence," *Journal of the American College of Cardiology,* Vol 53 No 11, pages 936-46.

11 Tibbits, op cit, page 75.

12 Tibbits, D, et al (2006), "Hypertension reduction through forgiveness training," *Journal of Pastoral Care & Counseling,* Vol 60 No 1-2, pages 27-34.

13 Chapman, G (2007), *Anger: Handling a Powerful Emotion in a Healthy Way,* Northfield Publishing, Chapter 3, pages 33-51.

14 Prochaska, J O, and C C DiClemente (1984), *The Transtheoretical Approach: Towards a Systematic Eclectic Framework,* Dow Jones Irwin.

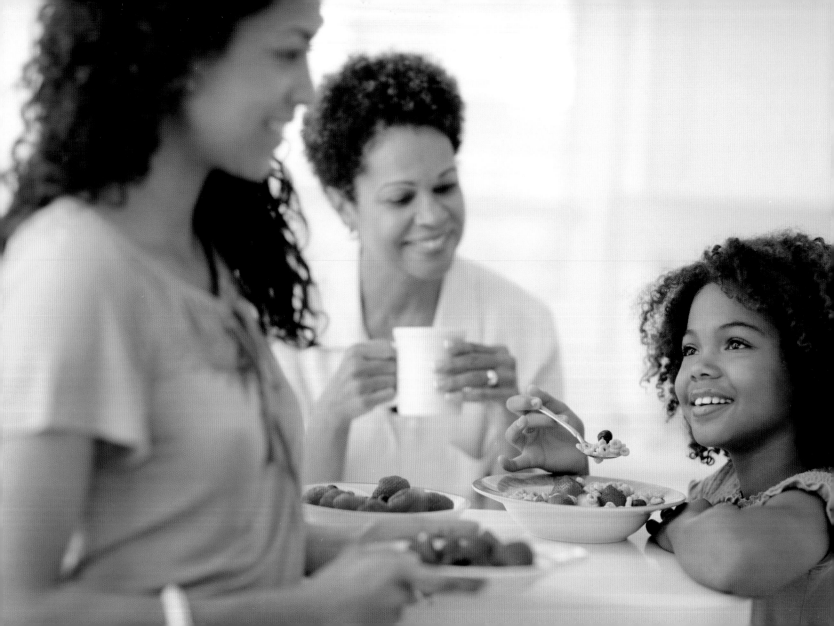

Chapter Fourteen

Your DNA is Not Your Destiny

Whenever we begin talking about lifestyle medicine, and the remarkable and proven difference that life-style choices can make to our health and wellbeing, inevitably someone will raise the question of genes. Usually with an air of resignation, they might say something like, "That sounds wonderful, but I simply have bad genes. My grandparents had this condition and my parents, too. So now I've got it as well."

Genetic factors and family history are important to keep in mind when considering risk factors for disease. But their direct impact on our health might not be as significant as many of us assume.

Researchers have found that as little as 30 per cent of our health outcomes are determined by issues outside of our control, including available medical care, environmental impacts and our DNA. This means our lifestyle—based on choices largely within our control—influences the remaining 70 per cent of our health.[1]

When it might seem that a disease or condition runs in the family, we need to remember that we do not only inherit our genes from our parents, we also inherit their lifestyle. Habits, traditions, attitudes and even recipes are passed from one generation to the next, forming a lifestyle that can have a greater health impact than many genetic predispositions.

This means our lifestyle-based on choices largely within our control-influences the remaining 70 per cent of our health.

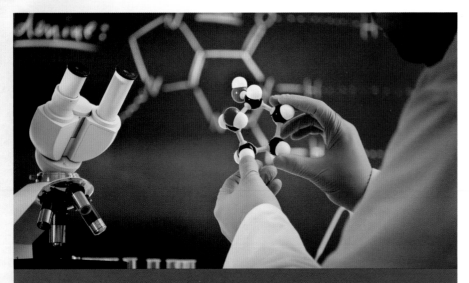

UNTANGLING DNA

Stretched end to end, the DNA in each cell in our body is almost 10 feet (3 meters) long. It contains about 30,000 separate genes, with thousands more variations. Some of the variations cause disease, like sickle cell anemia. Just one base-pair difference—just one mistake in the 3 billion parts—causes sickle cell disease.

But the vast majority of the variations are "silent" variations and do not cause any problem. This is how DNA testing can tell us apart. When conducting DNA testing, the technician is looking for the individual variations between us. It's more discriminating than fingerprints.

Introducing epigenetics

In January, 2010, *Time* magazine's cover story explained "Why your DNA isn't your destiny," introducing the new science of "epigenetics" and how it reveals that the choices we make change our genes.[2] Of course, we cannot change our DNA sequence but we can change how our genes work—and potentially how those of our children work.

The story begins in the 1960s when Francis Crick, James Watson and Maurice Wilkins received the 1962 Nobel Prize in Physiology or Medicine for their discovery that DNA was the "molecule of inheritance." Then, at the beginning of this century, Dr Francis Collins and his team on the Human Genome Project sequenced the entire human genome, identifying about 3 billion base pairs.

As we might recall from high school biology classes, we all come from two cells—one from our mother and one from our father. Each of those cells is incomplete, having only half of a set of 23 chromosomes. When joined together in the process of fertilization, they form a cell with a complete set of 23 paired chromosomes. This completed cell lodges in the mother's uterus and begins to grow, doubling and tripling, until there are trillions of cells.

This means that every cell in our body has a copy of that first full set of 23 chromosomes and the 30,000 genes they contain, whether part of our ear, toe or brain matter. To make a working body of all these identical but differently functioning cells, the majority of the genes in every cell are turned off. So rather than the genes themselves, the more significant difference in how cells work is the combinations formed by turning genes on and off during the cells' development. This is the real process that makes us the unique organisms that we are.

These discoveries dramatically change our understanding of lifestyle and genes. Though we often think of it that way, we do not actually inherit DNA from our parents. Rather, we inherit chromosomes, which are only 50 per cent DNA.[3]

The other 50 per cent of the chromosomes is made up of protein molecules, which also carry important information.

Inside the cell nucleus, the chromosomes are unraveled and made ready to be used. It takes a lot of nano-machinery inside each cell to turn those switches on and off. The protein molecules contain the switches.

And the most powerful way to change the switch setting is something simple: eating. The scientific research so far reveals that nutrition changes more switch settings than anything else discovered. A whole field of study—called nutrigenomics—has developed, seeking to discover which nutrients turn which genes on and off. It's turning out to be far more complicated than we initially imagined because it seems a single nutrient can switch a number of genes on or off, not just one.[4] It's more like conducting an orchestra than playing an individual instrument.

The most powerful way to change the switch setting is something simple: eating. The scientific research so far reveals that nutrition changes more switch settings than anything else discovered.

Switching genes off

The mother's diet changed the switch settings in the baby before it was born in ways that could be seen easily after birth.

A few years ago researchers did an experiment to test what could be done with diet to affect the genes.[5] This study looked at Agouti mice fed a tailored diet—designed to turn off the mice's special genes—during pregnancy to see what impact this would have on the genes in the baby.

The Agouti mouse is a unique mouse because it has been specially modified genetically to have the genes that cause obesity, heart disease and diabetes—all the chronic diseases afflicting so many people around the world—so they can be studied in a mouse model. One advantage of this kind of research is that mouse generations occur much faster than human generations.

The researchers were specifically interested in whether they could do something to alter the effects of the mouse's special genes and whether this would have any effect on future generations.

When the baby was born to this mother mouse that had been fed the special diet, the results were remarkable and dramatically changed scientific thinking. The baby didn't even look like the mother and didn't have the distinctive fur color that had been engineered to identify these mice. DNA testing of the baby mouse revealed the same genes for disease as those engineered into its mother, but they had been silenced—they were turned "off" in the womb.[6]

The mother's diet changed the switch settings in the baby before it was born in ways that could be seen easily after birth. The researchers further observed that the effects were evident for "three to four generations." This sounds amazing but remember the mother's egg is formed in her ovaries during the first few months of fetal development in her mother's womb, meaning that part of what becomes us is formed in our grandmother's womb.

Sometimes we forget the connectedness that we have between generations and the impact our choices can have on later generations.

Switching genes on

Another study focused on the impact of feeding a high-fat diet to pregnant rats.[7] The diet consisted of 50 per cent fat, similar to some meals that can be purchased at many fast-food restaurants.

Researchers were able to identify a gene on chromosome 3 in the developing fetus that was being over-expressed. The mother's high-fat diet was causing this gene to be turned on more than it should be, producing anatomical changes in the brain of the developing baby. More neurons were being produced than would normally have been, and these neurons were located in the base of the developing brain, where they became hormonally active.

This mother's diet produced an increase in hormonally active cells in the brain of her developing baby. When the offspring reached adolescence, these cells produced hormones that caused the growing rat to have high blood lipids—cholesterol and triglycerides—and higher food intake. This adolescent also preferred fatty foods, if given the choice compared to a regular diet. Researchers observed that the offspring had early onset of puberty and higher body weight.

We are seeing a similar result replicated in many developed nations today. For example, pediatricians in the United States are now advised to begin screening children for high cholesterol levels at age two, and begin statin medications by age eight.

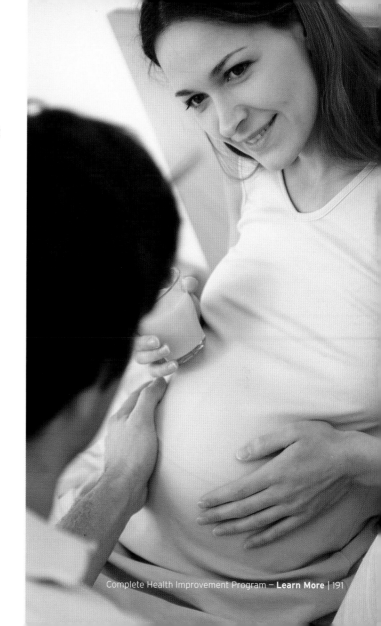

The differences between identical twins

Monozygotic twins—also known as identical twins—are essentially clones. They both came from the single fertilized cell, which separated into two parts sometime during the first few days after fertilization—maybe even during the first few hours. At this early stage of development, each part is capable of becoming a separate and complete human being. Because they carry the same genes, identical twins provide a unique opportunity to study epigenetic effects on gene expression during normal life. We all know that while identical twins are remarkably similar, they are also different—and their differences become more pronounced as they grow older.

Researchers have examined the degree of gene expression and epigenetic differences in identical twins over their lifetimes.[8] They compared the degree of difference at three years of age to the amount of difference at 50 years of age in 80 sets of identical twins.

Remarkably, they found as many as 1200 differences in gene expression in the three-year-old twins. Even though these identical twins shared many experiences and environmental exposures, there were differences in their lives that affected their respective gene expression. Not surprisingly then, they found much larger differences in gene expression in the 50-year-old twins, with more than 5500 genes expressed differently. Careful analysis revealed that the differences in gene expression correlated with measureable differences in the epigenome or, as we have learned, the epigenetic mechanisms and "protein switches" that modulate gene expression.

This research shows that gene expression is controlled more by epigenetic changes than by DNA sequence, since each of the monozygotic twin pairs studied shared the same DNA sequence. Our lifestyle choices likely exert stronger effects on gene expression than does the DNA we inherited. This is great news because we cannot do much about the DNA sequence we inherited, but we can do plenty about the lifestyle choices we make each and every day.

Even though these identical twins shared many experiences and environmental exposures, there were differences in their lives that affected their respective gene expression.

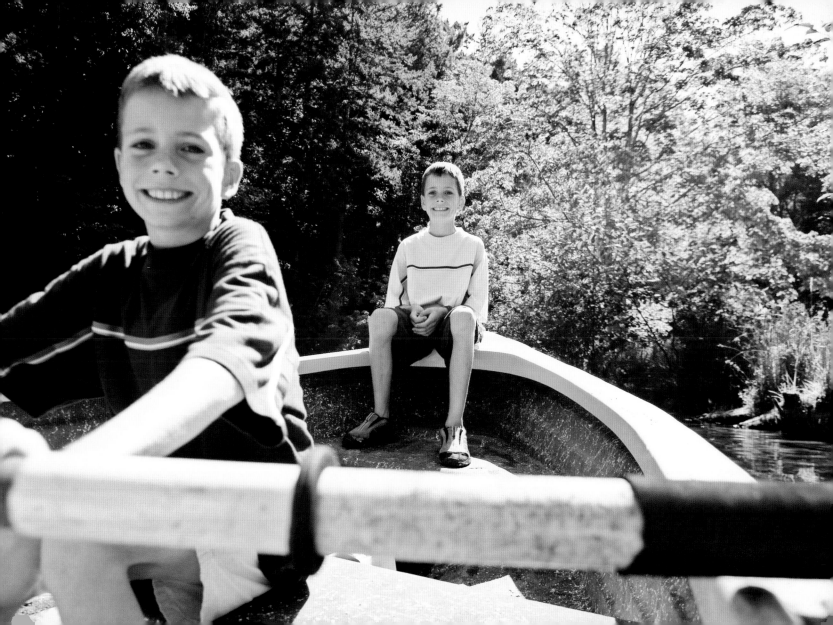

The conclusions: You have a choice!

One of the researchers who was part of the team who started this area of study when working with the Agouti mouse, Dr Jirtle explained the difference their results have made to our understanding of the interaction between our genes and health: "Epigenetics is proving we have some responsibility for the integrity of our genome. Before, genes predetermined outcomes. Now everything we do–everything we eat or smoke–can affect our gene expression and that of future generations. Epigenetics introduces the concept of free will into our idea of genetics."[9]

This is important to our understanding of lifestyle medicine and the real benefits we can enjoy from choosing an optimal lifestyle. The genetic objection is no longer valid. We do not have to think of ourselves as victims of our inheritance. Our lifestyle choices can alter even the effects of our genes.

Dr Feinberg of Johns Hopkins University urges that "epigenetics is at the epicenter of modern medicine."[10] Epigenetics helps explain the relationship between an individual's genetic background, the environment, aging and disease. This area of research is likely to grow in significance in our understanding of lifestyle medicine and genetics.

It's another significant reason that optimal lifestyle choices can change our lives:

> Change your diet and lifestyle, and it changes your epigenome.

> Change the epigenome and it changes your gene expression.

> Change your gene expression and it changes you–literally causing your body to be different.

Though we cannot change the DNA sequence, we may be able to change whether the genes are turned on or off. More of our health is within our control.

"Everything we do–everything we eat or smoke–can affect our gene expression and that of future generations."

KEY POINTS

> Epigenetics is a complicated and growing field of scientific research that offers further evidence of the importance of healthy lifestyle choices.

> While our genetic heritage plays a role in our health risks, so do lifestyle-related family habits and practices. Researchers suggest some 70 per cent of our health and wellbeing is determined by lifestyle factors that generally result from our everyday choices.

> While we inherit DNA from our parents, the most significant influence on how these genes are turned on or off in our body is our nutrition—what we do or do not eat.

Chapter Fourteen References

1   Danaei, G, et al (2009), "The preventable causes of death in the United States: comparative risk assessment of dietary, lifestyle, and metabolic risk factors," PLoS Medicine, Vol 6 No 4, e1000058.

2   Cloud, J (2010), "Why Your DNA Isn't Your Destiny," Time, January 6, 2010, <www.time.com/time/magazine/article/0,9171,1952313,00.html#ixzz24POuVP6g>; see also Ethan Watters, "DNA is not Destiny," Discover Magazine, Nov 2006, <www.geneimprint.com/media/pdfs/1162334912_fulltext.pdf>.

3   Emma Whitelaw interviewed about epigenetics by Fiona Wylie (2009), "Nature or Nurture? Neither!" Australian Life Scientist, November/December 2009 issue, <www.lifescientist.com.au/article/330686/feature_nature_nurture_neither_/>.

4   Kaput. J (2004), "Diet-disease gene interactions," Nutrition, Vol 20, pages 26-31; Gallou-Kabani, C, et al (2007), "Nutri-epigenomics: Lifelong remodeling of our epigenomes by nutritional and metabolic factors and beyond," Clinical Chemistry and Laboratory Medicine, Vol 45 No 3, pages 321-7.

5   Wolff, G, et al (1998), "Maternal epigenetics and methyl supplementation affect agouti gene expression in Avy/a mice," Journal of the Federation of American Societies for Experimental Biology, Vol 12 No 11, pages 949-57.

6   Waterland, R, and R Jirtle (2004), "Early nutrition, epigenetic changes at transposons and imprinted genes, and enhanced susceptibility to adult chronic diseases," Nutrition, Vol 20 No 1, pages 63-8.

7   Guo-Qing Chang, et al (2008), "Maternal High-Fat Diet and Fetal Programming: Increased proliferation of hypothalamic peptide-producing neurons that increase risk for overeating and obesity," The Journal of Neuroscience, Vol 28 No 46, pages 12107-19.

8   Fraga, M, et al (2005), "Epigenetic differences arise during the lifetime of monozygotic twins," Proceedings of the National Academy of Sciences, Vol 102 No 30, pages 10604-9.

9   Waterland and Jirtle, op cit.

10 Feinberg, A (2008), "Epigenetics at the center of modern medicine," Journal of the American Medical Association, Vol 299 No 11, pages 1345-50.

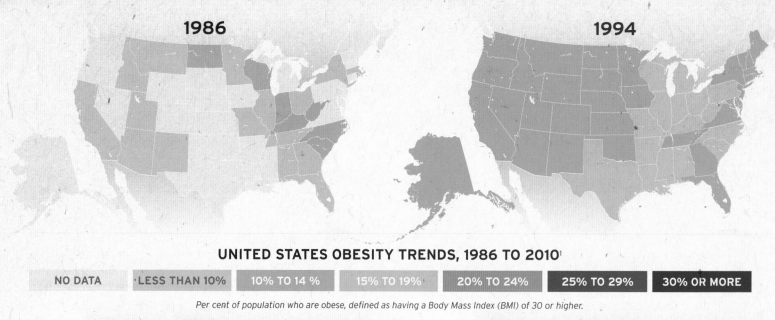

1986

1994

UNITED STATES OBESITY TRENDS, 1986 TO 2010[1]

| NO DATA | LESS THAN 10% | 10% TO 14 % | 15% TO 19% | 20% TO 24% | 25% TO 29% | 30% OR MORE |

Per cent of population who are obese, defined as having a Body Mass Index (BMI) of 30 or higher.

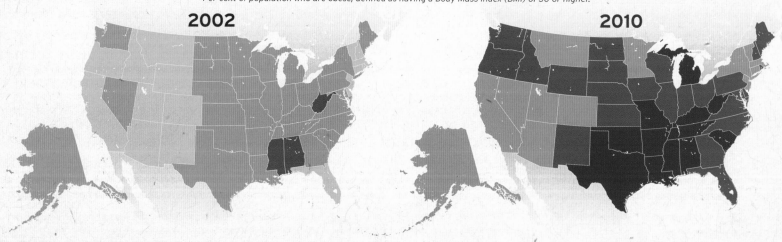

2002

2010

Chapter Fifteen

Re-engineer Your Environment

For the first time in history, more people are dying from the ill-effects of being overweight than under-weight.[2] About two-thirds of the world's population now lives in countries where being overweight or obese kills more people than malnutrition! Clearly we have a major crisis on our hands—an obesity epidemic—and what makes it so alarming is that obesity is linked to numerous conditions such as heart disease and musculoskeletal disorders, and it explains nearly half of type 2 diabetes cases.[3] And the more extra weight an individual is carrying, the higher their risk of developing several cancers.[4]

The obesity epidemic seems to have begun in earnest in the 1980s when epidemiologists began to note significant increases in the "weight of the nation,"[5] as evidenced by the United States obesity maps from the Centers for Disease Control (opposite). Similarly, obesity has more than doubled globally since 1980.[6]

Living in an obesogenic environment

Obesity has many contributing factors. It is commonly thought that obesity is "in our genes" but while some people are more predisposed than others to gaining weight—as we have seen—our genes are not our fate. Obviously, no-one becomes obese if they don't eat! As has been said before, "our genes load the gun, but our lifestyle pulls the trigger." The human genome has not changed enough during the past generation to explain the dramatic rise in obesity.

Another common misunderstanding is that obesity is related to a character flaw or weakness. Too often, overweight individuals are labeled as

About two-thirds of the world's population now lives in countries where being overweight or obese kills more people than malnutrition!

Our modern environment supports obesity—it is "obesogenic."

"gluttons" or "lazy" but this is inaccurate and unfair. Many thin people have no more ability to control their food intake and are not partial to moving if they don't have to!

Basic physiology tells us fat is simply excess energy, so the rise of obesity is a sign that collectively we are eating too much energy-dense food and not moving enough. But one reason this has become easier to do is that our modern environment enables or even encourages it.[7]

For most of us living in the developed world, food is plentiful and accessible, especially highly processed, fattening food. Not only is it available at every turn, we are strongly encouraged to consume it through clever marketing, strategic product placement and the fact that "everyone else is doing it." At the same time we are surrounded by labor-saving devices to make life easier and less energy demanding for us, which results in us moving less. Our modern environment supports obesity—it is "obesogenic."

So if you struggle with your weight, it is not all your fault. Many of the ill-health conditions we see in our society can be contributed to by our environment working against us.

But here is the good news: becoming aware of the influence your environment has on your lifestyle habits allows you to do something about it. A critical part of the solution to combating the obesity epidemic—as well as many of the other health problems facing us today—lies in re-engineering our environment to enable and encourage us to make healthier lifestyle choices. If we do this re-engineering well, we can even set up an environment in which healthy choices become our default and we make them even without thinking. So let's reflect on some of the dimensions of our environment:

› Political and economic factors

Economics can have perverse effects. One of the best examples of this can be seen in the history of the smoking industry. By the 1960s, smoking rates were declining within the medical community as the evidence accumulated that smoking increased the risk of cancer. Yet while doctors largely abandoned tobacco, misleading advertisements helped secure a rise in its use among their patients.[8]

Even now there is overwhelming evidence that smoking is deadly, tobacco companies still work to increase their sales. And their efforts have been so successful that even after their deceptions have been exposed, some still doubt that nicotine is addictive or that tobacco is harmful.[9] Subsequent lawsuits have discovered internal documents revealing that tobacco executives knew science had shown nicotine to be addictive and had paid researchers to publish studies designed to confuse the evidence and thwart efforts to regulate tobacco products. Alarmingly, research is showing that even so-called "tobacco education programs" are used to market tobacco products to potential young consumers.[10]

UNINTENDED CONSEQUENCES

The food processing industry provides thousands of valuable jobs and is a key contributor to the United States economy. Many financial incentives at a political level support processed foods, but the reasons for this can be complicated and don't necessarily align with our healthcare needs. For example, while public health officials in the United States promote "5 a Day"—consuming five or more servings of fruits and vegetables each day—as well as other campaigns to increase consumption of fruits and vegetables, government subsidies for processed foods far outweigh those for the foods we should consume more of. Incredibly, US crop subsidies in 2010 provided more financial support for tobacco than for the crops needed to supply the five or more servings of fruits and vegetables![11]

Approximate subsidies for food crops, 1996 to 2010[12]

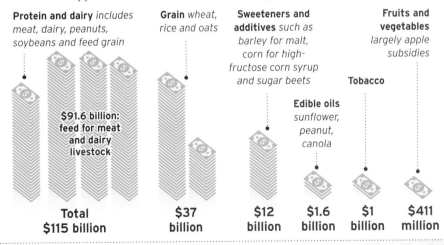

Protein and dairy *includes meat, dairy, peanuts, soybeans and feed grain*

$91.6 billion: feed for meat and dairy livestock

Total $115 billion

Grain *wheat, rice and oats*

$37 billion

Sweeteners and additives *such as barley for malt, corn for high-fructose corn syrup and sugar beets*

$12 billion

Edible oils *sunflower, peanut, canola*

$1.6 billion

Tobacco

$1 billion

Fruits and vegetables *largely apple subsidies*

$411 million

THOSE ADVERTISING BUDGETS

As if hyper-palatable, highly processed foods are not appealing enough, huge sums of money are spent encouraging us to eat more of them through clever advertising—much of which is aimed at children to groom their behaviors from early in life. According to the World Health Organization, "research shows that food advertising geared to children is extensive, that a significant amount of the marketing is for foods with a high content of fat, sugar or salt, and that television advertising influences children's food preferences, purchase requests and consumption patterns."[13]

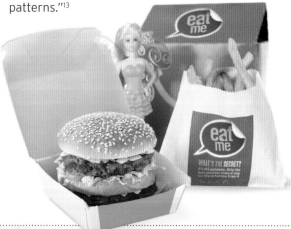

The story of the smoking industry is a clear example that economics, which can drive politics, can have a powerful effect on the environment we find ourselves in. Tragically, smoking still remains one of the leading causes of death in the world.[14] In some ways, we could compare this example to the rise of processed foods. It is in a food manufacturer's best financial interest, whether they produce healthy or unhealthy food, to sell more product to make greater profits.

Few people realize the extent to which processed, manufactured foods have been designed to increase consumption.[15] If food manufacturers want to sell more product, it is in their best interest to make the food as appealing as possible, be that by making it taste better, cost less or be convenient to eat.[16]

There is nothing inherently wrong with this. For example, your local fruit and vegetable market uses some of these tactics to a lesser extent when trying to sell you healthy plant foods. They display the choicest fruit in appealing patterns and highlight the in-season bargains of the week, all with the aim of getting you to buy more.

While ever these practices of food production and promotion exist, we need to be aware of them and take personal responsibility for the foods we choose. While not all processed foods are inherently unhealthy, unhealthy processed foods are always going to exist and it is in the financial best interests of some companies to sell them. If we are aware of this and aware of the power that good food choices can have on our health, we are one step closer to re-engineering our environment.[17]

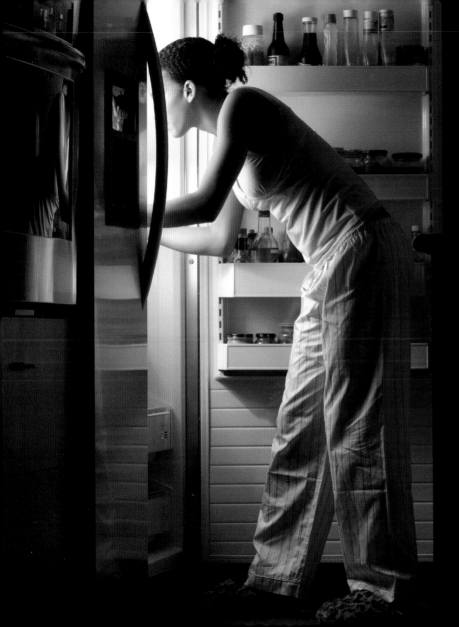

FOOD ADDICTION?

Brain scans reveal our brain reacts much the same to hyper-palatable foods as it does to cocaine and other habit-forming substances and practices.[18] In other words, hyper-palatable foods trigger the same brain circuitry involved in other addictions and cessation after habitual consumption of such foods can produce withdrawal-type symptoms.

Research reveals this is what sugar, fat and salt can do. Animals will work for such foods, even when they are not hungry, and seek out locations where they have found these foods previously. Of the three, sugar has been shown to have the strongest effects. However, a combination of two or more, especially sugar and fat, is stronger yet. Careful research by food scientists and neurochemists has found optimal concentrations to maximally stimulate the brain's pleasure centers, thus promoting overeating.[19]

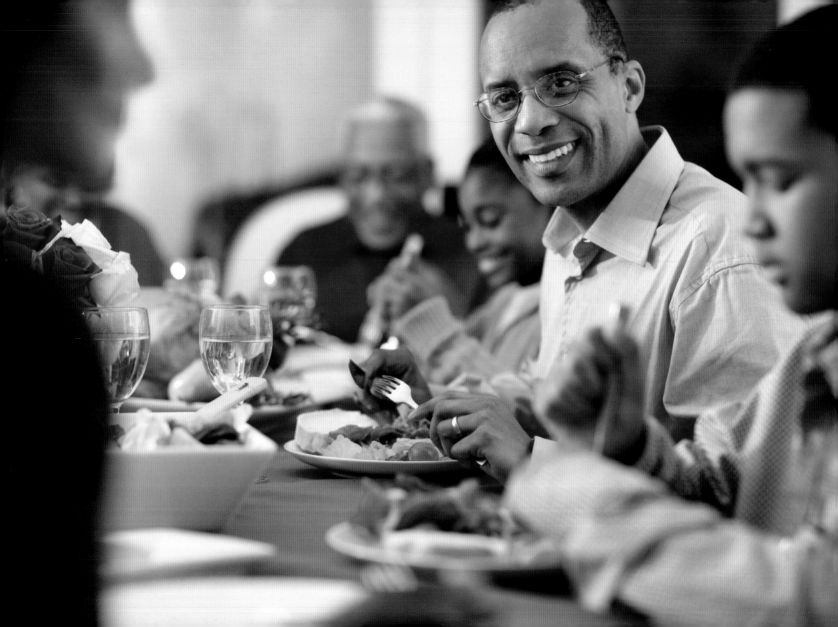

› Social environment

The "tribe" you belong to makes a huge difference to your health. Consider for example the fascinating results of a study by Harvard researchers.[20] The researchers tracked more than 12,000 individuals from the Framingham population for longer than 30 years. Their study found that an individual's likelihood of becoming obese increased by 37 per cent if their spouse became obese. However, if that individual had a friend who became obese, their chance of becoming obese increased by a staggering 171 per cent! This demonstrates the power of social influences to affect our weight—obviously genetics are not to blame in either of these instances. It also shows that mutual friends have a four- to five-times greater influence on each other than spouses.

Intriguingly, the researchers discovered that in social networks, an individual who gains weight increases the chance by about 10 per cent that the friends of their friends—three degrees of separation—will also gain weight. Obviously, obesity is a socially contagious condition and as such we need to address social issues if we are to overcome the obesity epidemic. The good news, however, is that the study also found the reverse was true—an individual who lost weight had a positive influence on their extended social network.

Obesity is socially contagious because our lifestyle practices tend to assimilate to those with whom we associate. This is especially the case in relation to food. Food is so ingrained in culture—we eat together, and use food to socialize and celebrate. While this is an important function of food, it can make it all the more difficult to make healthy food choices if everyone around is not interested. The same applies to physical activity. As society increasingly relies on social media for connecting and interacting, these social forces are responsible for transitioning people to more and more sedentary "screen time."

To set ourselves for success, we must be aware of the power of our social environment to affect our lifestyle choices and habits. Awareness allows us to plan ahead so we can better negotiate this powerful force. For instance, to maximize our success at maintaining a healthy eating pattern it might be helpful—even necessary—to decide on strategies to negotiate an unsupportive spouse or children who might not like what is on the menu at home.

When your existing social structures are not supportive, it can be helpful to add new ones. This is what CHIP is all about. Other examples include signing up for vegetarian cooking classes, joining a gym, or teaming up with a sporting club. Aligning and surrounding ourselves with others who share similar values and goals is crucial to re-engineering our environment to facilitate our journey to better health.

› Physical surroundings

The final aspect of our environment that has an extremely influential effect on our lifestyle habits is our physical surroundings. Consider physical activity, for example. One of the most effective ways to increase individuals' physical activity levels is providing them with easily accessible opportunities to be active, such as walking paths and cycle ways.[21] The same principle applies to food. If we have ready access to fast foods and nutritious foods are hard to come by, it is far more likely that we will make the poorer choice.

Our physical surroundings largely determine our default behaviors—what we do without thinking about it. If there are seats available on the train, we will tend to sit down. If there is a block of chocolate or jar of candy on our desk, we will tend to consume them almost subconsciously.

This provides us with an important insight: to make better lifestyle choices more consistently, we should re-engineer our physical environment so positive choices are the easy ones, and the not-so-good choices are more difficult. For the good choices to become our default, we need to create a situation where they are the most accessible, and if possible, the mandated behaviors. It is unrealistic to remove all the fast-food stores from your vicinity and shut down the lifts in your building so you are forced to take the stairs, but there are many things we can re-engineer within our personal sphere. For example, you can:

> Hide junk food, so you will not be drawn subconsciously to it every time it catches your eye. Better still, don't have it in your house.

> Purge your pantry. If overcome by a craving, you are less likely to cave in if the unhealthy food is not readily available.

> Set up your workspace so your phone is not near your chair, so you have to stand when speaking on the phone.

Our physical surroundings are tremendously influential on our lifestyle choices and habits, so it is important we carefully consider how we can surround ourselves with a physical environment conducive to positive lifestyle choices.

Our physical surroundings largely determine our default behaviors—what we do without thinking about it.

Making smarter choices

The choices we make and our ability to stick to them make all the difference.

The ability to motivate ourselves to do the things we don't really feel like but know we should—or refrain from doing the things we feel like, even though we know we shouldn't—is a core component of *emotional intelligence*. Emotional intelligence includes a variety of skills, but the ability to motivate oneself and delay gratification are key components.[22] Intriguingly, emotional intelligence is a good predictor of how "successful" an individual will be not just in their health but in many aspects of life, including their finances and relationships.

To live our best life calls for emotional intelligence skills, which are learnable and trainable. Exciting developments in our understanding of the brain have led to the concept of "brain plasticity." We now know that the brain can and does grow and change, depending on what we do with it. Every time we learn a new skill or practise a new behavior, we activate and strengthen pathways through our brain that make us better

at it: "Neurons that fire together, wire together."[23] As we practise new skills and behaviors, we become better at them—they become more automatic and easier for us to do.

We can get better at making good choices, too—if we practise them. We can practise making good choices like not putting ourselves in situations where physical or social cues make it difficult for us to follow through on our resolve to live healthier. Consciously avoiding high-risk situations is recognized as imperative for relapse prevention for those trying to break the chains of alcohol and other addictions.[24]

We can also practise making better choices regarding the "triggers" that spiral our behaviors out of control. Don't eat the first square of chocolate if you know it will lead to eating the entire block!

We can practise making better choices when we are faced with cravings for the things that are not helpful to us. Each positive choice strengthens our resolve and grows our ability to make better choices in the future.

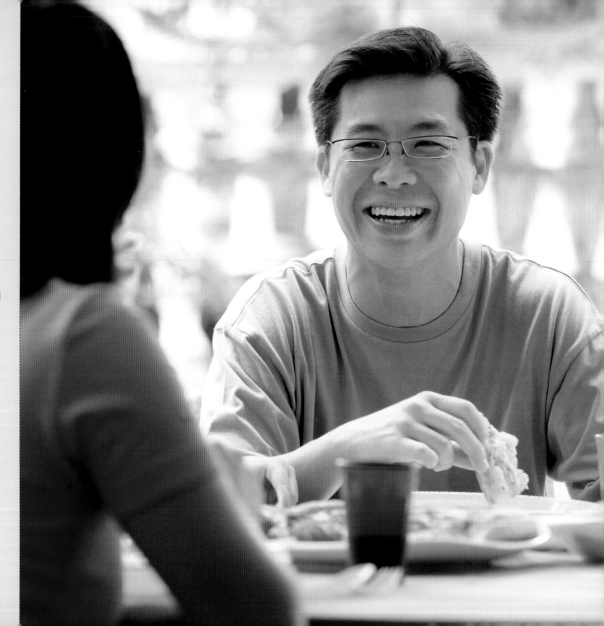

KEY POINTS

> Without us even being aware of it, our environment can have a profound effect on our lifestyle choices and our wellbeing. Our "environment" includes the political and economic climate we live in, the social influences we are exposed to and our physical surroundings.

> To set ourselves up for success in living a healthier lifestyle, we should endeavor to engineer our environment so it supports healthier lifestyle habits.

> Resourced with a supportive environment, it is also important that we practise and develop the skill of making positive lifestyle choices.

Chapter Fifteen References

1   Center for Disease Control and Prevention (2011), "Overweight and Obesity–Obesity Trends Among U.S. Adults Between 1985 and 2010." < http://www.cdc.gov/obesity/downloads/obesity_trends_2010.pdf>

2   World Health Organization (2011), "Obesity Fact Sheet," No 311, <www.who.int/mediacentre/factsheets/fs311/en/index.html>.

3   ibid.

4   World Cancer Research Fund Expert Report (2007), "Food, nutrition, physical activity, and the prevention of cancer: a global perspective," <www.wcrf.org>.

5   Flegal, K M, et al (1998), "Overweight and obesity in the United States: prevalence and trends, 1960-1994," International Journal of Obesity Related Metabolic Disorders, Vol 22 No 1, pages 39-47; Kuczmarski, R J, et al (1994), "Increasing Prevalence of Overweight Among US Adults–The National Health and Nutrition Examination Surveys, 1960 to 1991," Journal of the American Medical Association, Vol 272 No 3, pages 205-11.

6   WHO, op cit.

7   Swinburn, B, and G Egger (2004), "The runaway train: too many accelerators, not enough brakes," British Medical Journal, Vol 329, pages 736-9.

8   Smith, D R (2008), "The historical decline of tobacco smoking among United States physicians: 1949-1984," Tobacco Induced Diseases, Vol 4 No 9.

9   Glantz, S, et al (2008), "Tobacco industry sociological programs to influence public beliefs about smoking," Social Science and Medicine, Vol 66 No 4, pages 970-81.

10 Klesges, R C, et al (2009), "Do we believe the tobacco industry lied to us? Association with smoking behavior in a military population," Health Education Research, Vol 24 No 6, pages 909-21.

11 Environmental Working Group (2010), "Farm Subsidy Database, 2010," <http://farm.ewg.org/region.php?fips=00000&progcode=total&yr=2010>.

12 Environmental Working Group, USDA, EPA, Soybean Meal Infocenter, American Soybean Association, American Peanut Council. The Washington Post, October 3, 2011.

13 World Health Organization (2012), "Political Declaration of the High-level Meeting of the General Assembly on the Prevention and Control of Non-communicable Diseases. Sixty-sixth session, Agenda item 117," <www.who.int/nmh/events/un_ncd_summit2011/political_declaration_en.pdf>.

14 Mokdad, A H, et al (2004), "Actual Causes of Death in the United States, 2000," Journal of American Medical Association, Vol 291 No 10, pages 1238-45.

15 Kessler, D A (2009), The End of Overeating: Taking control of the insatiable American appetite, Rodale Press.

16 Pollan, M (2006), The Omnivore's Dilemma: A history of four meals, Penguin Press.

17 French, S, et al (2001), "Environmental influences on eating and physical activity," Annual Review of Public Health, Vol 22, pages 309-35.

18 Gaysinskaya, V A, et al (2011), "Hyperphagia induced by sucrose: relation to circulating and CSF glucose and corticosterone and orexigenic peptides in the arcuate nucleus," Pharmacology Biochemistry and Behavior, Vol 97 No 3, pages 521-30.

19 Kessler, op cit.

20 Christakis, N A, and J H Fowler (2007), "The Spread of Obesity in a Large Social Network over 32 Years," New England Journal of Medicine, Vol 357 No 4, pages 370-9.

21 Popkin, B, et al (2005), "Environmental influences on food choice, physical activity and energy balance," Physiology & Behavior, Vol 86, pages 603-13.

22 Goleman, D (1995), Emotional Intelligence. Why it can matter more than IQ, Bantam.

23 Doidge, N (2010), The Brain That Changes Itself: Stories of Personal Triumph from the Frontiers of Brain Science, Scribe, page 63.

24 Larimer, M, et al (1999), "Relapse Prevention: An Overview of Marlatt's Cognitive-Behavioral Model," Alcohol Research and Health, Vol 23 No 2, pages 151-60.

Section 5:

From Health to Happiness

We have focused primarily on the two pillars of lifestyle medicine—nutrition and physical activity—and how to remove roadblocks on the journey toward embracing them. However, whole person health is much like a jigsaw puzzle, with all pieces interconnected. While nutrition and physical activity are two important pieces, they do not make up the whole puzzle. In this final section, we turn our attention to discovering the secrets of living well as we move beyond health to happiness.

Chapter Sixteen looks at the evidence that our psychological state has a tremendous influence on our health and examines the reasons why, then considers positive strategies for managing stress.

Chapter Seventeen examines five strategies for improving your mood.

Chapter Eighteen explores the latest research and asks the question, "What does it take to truly flourish in life?"

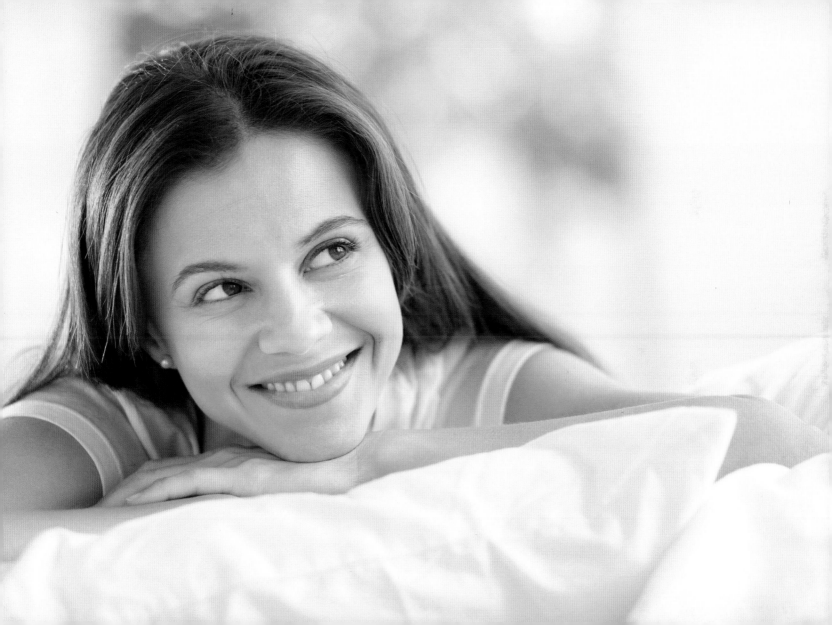

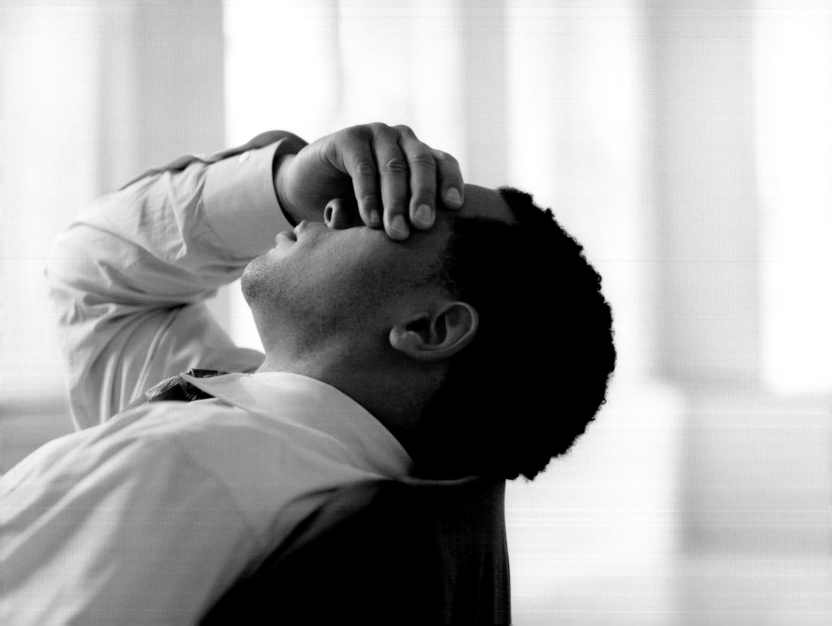

Chapter Sixteen

Stress-relieving Strategies

Imagine you are driving your car without a care in the world when suddenly you hear a siren. In your rear-view mirror, you see blue flashing lights and the driver of the vehicle indicating for you to pull over to the side of the road. You don't bother to glance down at your speedometer because you already know you were traveling too fast.

You can identify the changes that instantly occur in your body: racing pulse, sweaty palms, tense muscles, unsettled stomach and more. These symptoms are commonly referred to as the "stress response." While most people don't find them pleasant at the time, the stress response is designed to help us deal with emergency situations. Essentially it gears the body for "fight or flight." Neither response is recommended when being pulled over by the police, but they are appropriate if being pursued by something that wants to eat you.

While the stress response can serve us well in the moment, it is not helpful when constantly activated. The perils of a chronically activated stress response was first documented in 1956 by pioneer stress researcher, Dr Hans Selye, who noted that if the state of "alarm" created by the stress response persisted, it lead to a state of "exhaustion."[1]

Since that time, extensive research has demonstrated an association between ongoing stress and all manner of diseases, including diseases not traditionally thought of as stress-related. For example, there is emerging evidence that stress plays a part in diabetes,[2] which is not surprising given that one of the functions of the stress response is to alter the body's blood sugar level to equip us with more energy to escape the present danger.

Extensive research has demonstrated an association between ongoing stress and all manner of diseases, including diseases not traditionally thought of as stress-related.

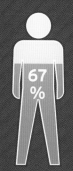

Stressed-out numbers[3]

Unfortunately, many people today have a chronically activated stress response, with work, family, finances and health being common contributors:

FINANCIAL STRESS

75 per cent of women compared to 67 per cent of men report that money is a significant source of stress in their life.

67 %

75 %

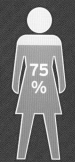

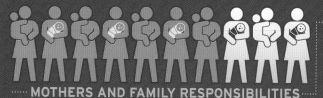

MOTHERS AND FAMILY RESPONSIBILITIES

• 7 out of 10 mothers report that family responsibilities are a significant source of stress.[4]

69 per cent of employees report that work is a significant source of stress.

• 41 per cent of employees say they typically feel tense or stressed out during the workday.

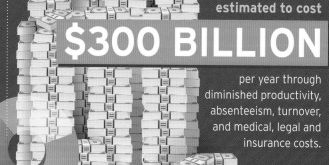

Workplace stress is estimated to cost

$300 BILLION

per year through diminished productivity, absenteeism, turnover, and medical, legal and insurance costs.

Why ongoing "distress" affects health and wellbeing

"Stress" commonly describes the negative emotional state we encounter when we feel overloaded. But this is a slight misuse of the term. Dr Selye defined "stress" as a response of the body to any demand for change and he pointed out that stress is necessary if we are to be our best. For example, exercise is a form of stress as it calls the body out of its mellow resting state, the outcome of which is a fitter, healthier body. In the same way, if we have nothing to get us out of bed in the morning, we are typically unproductive.

Indeed, we need some stress in our lives and Dr Selye referred to the ideal level of stress as "eustress." But when the pressures mount, we move beyond eustress to "distress" and this is what many people are experiencing, especially those who have seen more change in their lifetime than any other period in history. Alarmingly, such distress is implicated in serious health concerns.

Distress directly influences our physiology

As imagined in the earlier scenario, distress can cause immediate changes in our physical state. Some of these changes are noticeable but others occur without us realizing.

› The cardiovascular system

The stress response excites a cascade of communications between the brain and body referred to as the Hypothalamic-Pituitary-Adrenal (HPA) axis. One of the outcomes of this is the release of adrenaline, which has an instant impact on the cardiovascular system. Adrenaline causes our heart to feel like it is going to jump out of our chest after we get a fright. Adrenaline also causes our blood vessels to constrict, driving up our blood pressure and making our skin cold to touch.

While these responses are helpful in emergency situations, quickly delivering oxygen and nutrients to our muscles, they can also take their toll. Researchers from the University of Carolina found that individuals with higher anger scores were two and a half times more likely to experience a cardiac event.[5] Similarly, exposure to traffic has been found to increase the risk of a heart attack in the following hour by almost three times.[6]

While activation of the stress response in the short-term can present problems, the greater danger lies when it is activated in the long term. In the INTERHEART study, which traced factors that contributed to the heart attacks of more than 14,000 individuals from 52 countries, the researchers found that an individual's psychosocial state was a more important determinant than their physical activity level or how many serves of fruit and vegetables they consumed daily.[7] There are probably many mechanisms responsible for this, but psychological distress is known to alter the "thickness" of the blood, as well as its clotting properties.[8]

Exposure to traffic has been found to increase the risk of a heart attack in the following hour by almost three times.

A WINDOW INSIDE

The first set of experiments to highlight the impact of emotions on gut function were conducted by Dr William Beaumont in the early part of the 19th century on an unfortunate subject by the name of Alexis St Martin.[9] Alexis had no intention of becoming a science experiment but when he was shot in the stomach, the wound healed in such a way that there was a hole leading from the inside of his stomach to the outside world. This hole allowed excellent viewing for Dr Beaumont to literally watch what goes on during the processes of digestion and he conducted more than 100 experiments on Alexis. Alexis tired of the experiments he was made to participate in by the higher authorities in the army in which he was serving and, when he became annoyed, Dr Beaumont observed that the lining of his stomach become inflamed. These observations first demonstrated that one's emotional state influences gut function and the processes of digestion.

Photograph of Alexis St. Martin

› Gut function

Distress is implicated in numerous gastrointestinal symptoms, including heartburn, indigestion, nausea and vomiting, diarrhea and constipation.[10] These conditions can present serious concerns as the gut is increasingly being recognized as an incredibly important organ. The lining of our intestine has a surface area more than 100 times that of our skin and our gut is home to about 100 trillion bacteria—10 times more than the number of cells in our body![11]

There is also developing awareness of an intimate connection between the brain and the gut, such that the state of our gut can influence the state of our brain. As 70 to 80 per cent of our immune cells are contained in gut-associated lymphoid tissue,[12] it is little wonder that an unhappy gastrointestinal system—as occurs when we are distressed—can powerfully affect our immune system.

› Immune function

Since George Solomon coined the term *psycho-neuro-immunology* in 1964,[13] the concept that our psychological state can affect our nervous

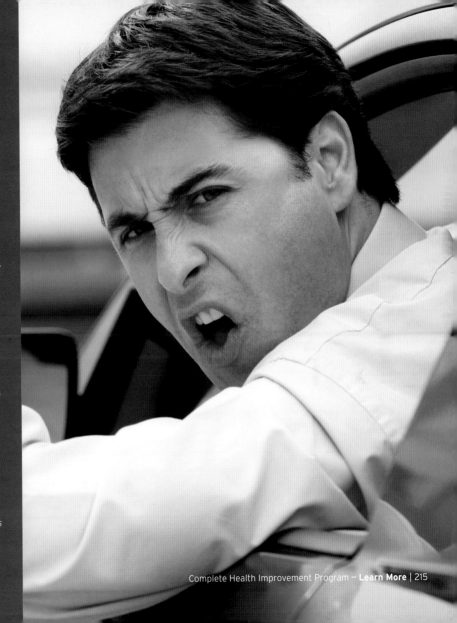

HOSTILITY AND HEALING

In one fascinating study, couples volunteered to take part in a "wound-healing" study. On two occasions separated by a couple of weeks, a standardized wound was administered to the forearm of each person using a suction device that created a blister. Following the "wounding," they participated in a counseling session with a trained therapist.

On one of the occasions, the therapist asked questions that promoted discussion about feel-good topics, such as their first date or wedding day. On the other occasion, the facilitator initiated conflict by asking about contentious issues, such as "Do you feel he communicates well with you?" and "How do you feel about her spending habits?"

Following the sessions, researchers monitored how long it took for the blister wounds to heal. They found that after the heated, angst-evoking "discussion," the wounds took as much as 30 per cent longer to heal.[14] The couples who really got into the spirit of the study and demonstrated a high level of hostility took 40 per cent longer to heal than the lower-hostility couples!

These findings are consistent with another study involving dental students in which wounds sustained three days before a major test healed on average 40 per cent slower than those made during the lower-stress summer vacation.[15]

Dangers of Distress

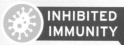

INHIBITED IMMUNITY

Our psychological state can affect our nervous system, that in turn affects our immune system.

Greater fear or distress prior to surgery is associated with poorer outcomes, including longer hospital stays, more post-operative complications, and higher rates of re-hospitalization.

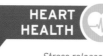

HEART HEALTH

Stress releases adrenaline, which increases our heart rate, causes our blood vessels to constrict, alters the "thickness" of our blood as well as its clotting properties, driving up our blood pressure, and makes our skin cold to touch.

EMOTIONAL EFFECTS

The stress response changes the way we feel, impacting our lifestyle choices. Distressed individuals are more likely to sleep poorly, have a greater propensity for alcohol and drug abuse, suffer food cravings causing poor nutrition choices, be impatient and lack the desire for exercise.

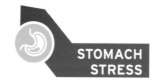

STOMACH STRESS

Distress can cause heartburn, indigestion, nausea and vomiting, diarrhea and constipation.

There is also a connection between the brain and the gut, such that the state of our gut can influence the state of our brain.

system, that in turn affects our immune system has progressed into an established science. Cortisol—the main stress hormone produced by activation of the stress response—inhibits the immune system. If the stress response persists for only a short time, this is not a serious concern, but if chronically activated it can lead to all manner of health problems.

Studies have repeatedly demonstrated that our psychological state influences the likelihood of getting sick. In a study in which volunteers were inoculated with several different strains of cold viruses, the best predictor of whether the individual would develop symptoms was the number and severity of the stressors they had faced during the previous month. And if you are unwell, your psychological state will influence how long it takes to get better. Greater fear or distress prior to surgery is associated with poorer outcomes, including longer hospital stays, more post-operative complications, and higher rates of re-hospitalization.[16]

How you *feel* effects how you *heal*.

Clearly, emotional distress can have a tremendous bearing on our health and wellbeing by directly influencing our physiology and the effects of stress go beyond the cardiovascular, gastrointestinal and immune systems. Cortisol has numerous effects, including weakening the skin and causing fat to be deposited around our center, which is the most dangerous form of obesity. But distress can also affect our health by altering our behavior in ways that sabotage our health and wellbeing.

Distress influences behaviors that effect our health

Have you ever resolved to eat healthier and done well until some stressful event came along? Suddenly your resolve weakened and you found comfort by gorging on all the things you had determined to avoid. Or have you made a commitment to get fit—perhaps even joining a gym—but the pressures of life mounted and your enthusiasm waned?

Our emotional state can have a profound effect on our behavior. The part of our brain responsible for how we feel is also the part of the brain responsible for our drives. Ask someone why they don't exercise and they are likely to say they

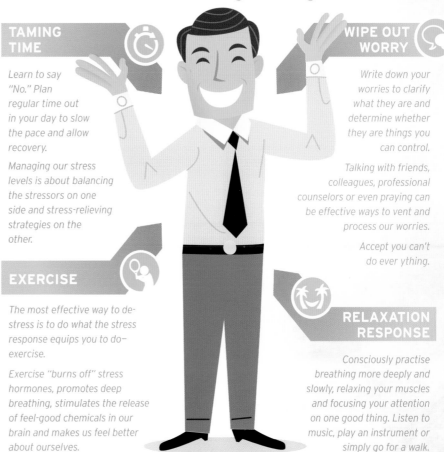

Stress-relieving Strategies

TAMING TIME

Learn to say "No." Plan regular time out in your day to slow the pace and allow recovery.

Managing our stress levels is about balancing the stressors on one side and stress-relieving strategies on the other.

WIPE OUT WORRY

Write down your worries to clarify what they are and determine whether they are things you can control.

Talking with friends, colleagues, professional counselors or even praying can be effective ways to vent and process our worries.

Accept you can't do everything.

EXERCISE

The most effective way to de-stress is to do what the stress response equips you to do—exercise.

Exercise "burns off" stress hormones, promotes deep breathing, stimulates the release of feel-good chemicals in our brain and makes us feel better about ourselves.

RELAXATION RESPONSE

Consciously practise breathing more deeply and slowly, relaxing your muscles and focusing your attention on one good thing. Listen to music, play an instrument or simply go for a walk.

don't *feel* like it. Similarly, ask someone why they ate the entire block of chocolate and they will say they *felt* like it. Much of what we do is about a feeling. Because the stress response changes the way we feel, it can have a marked impact on our lifestyle choices. Distressed individuals are more likely to exhibit behaviors that put them at greater risk of ill health, including poorer sleep and a greater propensity for alcohol and drug abuse, in addition to the poorer nutrition and less exercise already mentioned.[17]

The stress response is so strongly linked to alterations in our behavior that they can serve as a good sign we are stressed, even when we might not recognize the symptoms of distress in ourselves. For example, difficultly falling asleep or waking in the middle of the night and not being able to fall back to sleep, sitting on the couch and resisting movement at all costs, being impatient with others, experiencing food cravings, or letting the house get unusually messy, can all be signs that our stress levels are rising. Managing distress begins with being aware that we are suffering from it, so it is useful to note the behavior changes accompanying our stress response.

The stress response is so strongly linked to alterations in our behavior that they can serve as a good sign we are stressed.

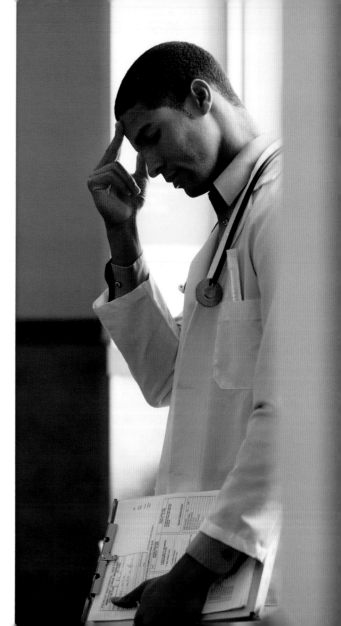

How to de-stress

Not everyone stresses to the same extent about the same things. For example, if we selected a random sample of individuals and stood them in front of an audience to tell a story, some would experience a stress response bordering on panic, while others would be relaxed and enjoy the experience. Stress is affected by such things as the circumstances, the personality of the individual, and his or her past experiences.

Yet, our stress levels are largely determined by the number and size of the stressors we face. If our stress levels are already high, a relatively small addition can tip us over the edge.

One strategy for managing our stress levels is to not place ourselves in a situation where we will confront too many stressors. Learning to say "no" can be helpful, especially when we already have a lot going on. And if we already have too much to do, it can be helpful to lighten the load. This might involve lowering your expectations of yourself—what you can achieve, acquire or become—as well as your expectations of others. Lowering our expectations of how much we need to achieve in a day can help slow the pace of life,

which can seem out of control for many people today. Archibald Hart, author of *Adrenaline and Stress,* describes stress as "hurry sickness" and asserts that part of the antidote involves planning regular time out to slow the pace and allow recovery.[18]

However, sometimes life seems out of control, throwing many stressors at us simultaneously. Having effective coping strategies is important. Managing our stress levels is about balancing the stressors on one side and stress-relieving strategies on the other. The greater our stressors, the greater our need for stress relief.

Coping strategies can be positive or negative. Negative coping strategies include alcohol abuse and drug use, as well as food and other addictions. Negative coping strategies do nothing to alleviate the stressors we are facing and they often create additional stressors. Fortunately, there are several positive techniques we can employ to tame the stress response.

Managing our stress levels is about balancing the stressors on one side and stress-relieving strategies on the other.

› Exercise

As already described, the stress response gears us up for "fight or flight," both of which are physically active pursuits. In *Why Zebras Don't Get Ulcers*,[19] Robert Sapolsky points out that when a zebra looks up and sees a lion bearing down on the herd, it experiences an immediate stress response. That stress response gears the zebra to either fight or take flight—presumably all living zebras opt for the latter.

Of course, there are two potential outcomes of the chase: the zebra gets caught or it gets away. In either instance, the zebra's stress response subsides quickly. Soon after the chase is called off, the zebra can be found going about its usual foraging and grazing. Dr Sapolsky notes that part of the reason the zebra can quickly return to a relaxed state is because the all-out sprint helps reset the stress response to baseline. In the same way, the stress response gets turned on to prepare humans for physical activity and one of the most effective ways to de-stress is to do what the stress response equips you to do—exercise.

The mechanisms by which exercise allows us to manage the stress response are not completely understood but they are likely to be multifaceted. For example, the stress benefits of exercise include:

> "Burning off" stress hormones.

> Promoting deep breathing, which can be therapeutic for relieving stress in its own right.

> Stimulating the release of feel-good chemicals in our brain.

> Making us feel better about ourselves.

> Providing us with an opportunity to step back from our stressors to gain clarity and identify potential ways to alleviate them.

Research indicates that exercise provides its best stress-reducing outcomes when it is taken regularly and higher intensities may be the most beneficial.

One of the most effective ways to de-stress is to do what the stress response equips you to do-exercise.

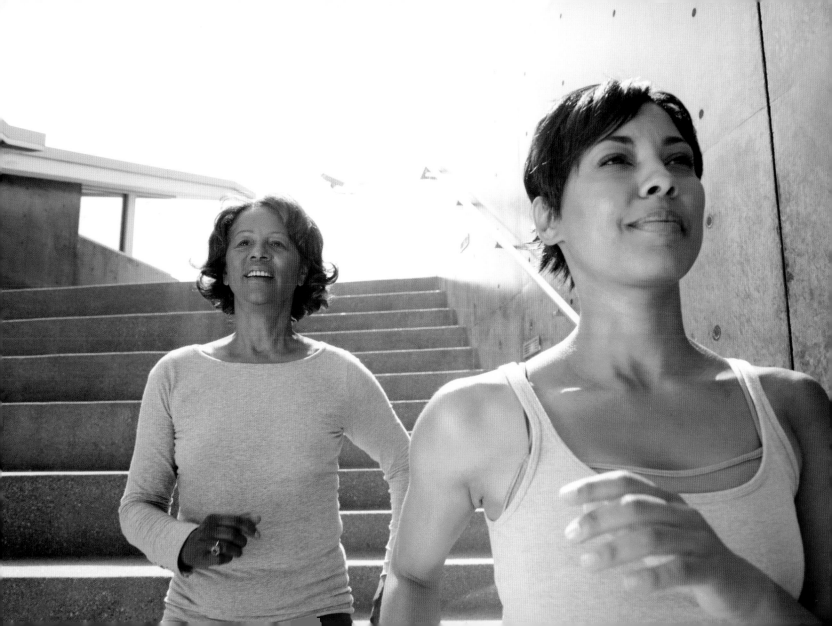

› Clarify your worries

"Humans are the only animals that create stress with their own minds," according to Dr Andrew Weil, director of the Integrative Medicine Program at the University of Arizona Medical School. "Managing stress has a lot to do with how we worry, and managing worry has a lot to do with where we focus our attention."[20]

Humans certainly have an incredible potential to create psychological stress through worry, arguably the greatest cause of suffering humans encounter. To return to the zebra, it seems unlikely that they wake up and think: "I wonder if the lions are hungry today. And I bet they are going to be hanging out at the watering hole that the herd will go to. And when they attack they are probably going to pick on me because my stripes are odd and make me stand out from the crowd! And I am sure my legs are shorter than everyone else's. I don't stand a chance! I'm a dead zebra walking! Ahhh!" Zebras don't catastrophize in that way–only humans do.

One useful strategy for gaining better clarity on our worries is to determine whether they are things we control. When our circle of concern is broader than our circle of influence, we set ourselves up for unproductive worry. By contrast, worries within our areas of control deserve appropriate action. Courageously dealing with them can be incredibly effective for bringing our stress levels down. Of course, the challenge often comes in knowing the difference between worries we can realistically do something about and those we cannot.

Writing your worries down can be extremely helpful in this regard. Once listed, apply the well-known wisdom of the "Serenity Prayer" to your catalogue of worries: "God grant me the serenity to accept the things I cannot change; the courage to change the things I can; and the wisdom to know the difference."

Another potentially powerful way to gain clarity and bring down the stress response is to talk with someone about your concerns. Dialoguing with friends, colleagues, professional counsellors or even praying can be effective ways to vent and process our worries.

Even if the listener doesn't offer wise advice, the act of talking it through can be what your brain needs to gain clarity on the situation. Talking it through can alert us to the fact that many of our worries are about unlikely events or risks. As Mark Twain once commented, "I have known a great many troubles, but most of them never happened."

› Practise the relaxation response

The relaxation response is a scientific strategy to reverse those symptoms of the stress response that we have conscious control over. While we don't have conscious control over our immune system or gut function, we can consciously practise breathing more deeply and slowly, relaxing our muscles and focusing our attention on one good thing. Reversing these symptoms of the stress response can be an extremely effective technique for dialing down the stress response and creating a state of calm.[21]

Here is a brief overview of the relaxation response, first popularized by pioneer researcher and author of *The Relaxation Response,* Dr Herbert Benson.[22] Before you start, it is important to set aside up to 20 minutes so you won't feel pressured or be interrupted:

› Sit or lie in a comfortable position, but your objective is not to fall asleep. As Hart notes, "Sleeping is not what relaxation is all about. . . . Relaxation is a conscious experience, not a trance or sleep-like state."[23]

› Think about each muscle in your body and completely relax them, starting at your feet and progressing up to your face. Once the muscles are relaxed, keep them relaxed. Sometimes an effective way to help a muscle relax is to contract it first, then "let go."

› Concentrate on your breathing. Take several slow, deep breaths through your nose, inflating the lower part of your diaphragm, then breathe naturally and easily.

› In this relaxed state, imagine being in a place that makes you feel calm and at peace—a deserted beach, high mountain peak or anywhere you feel relaxed and surrounded by beauty.

› Continue for 10 to 20 minutes. When you have finished, sit quietly—first with your eyes closed, then with your eyes open.

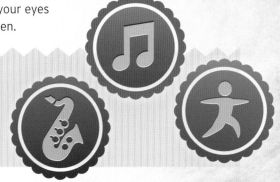

Dr Benson also suggests there are many other methods for achieving a relaxation response, including listening to music, playing an instrument, engaging in activities that require repetitive movements including repetitive aerobic exercise such as walking, and repeating affirming phrases. Regardless of the method used, daily practice can have a profound affect on our health and wellbeing.

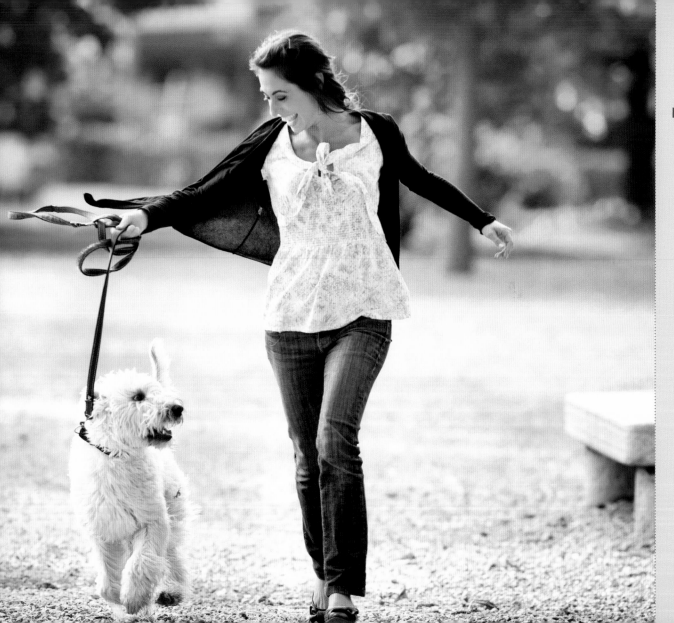

KEY POINTS

› Our psychological state has a tremendous impact on our health. It causes direct physiological changes and can also affect our health-related behaviors.

› One of the greatest causes of emotional distress is "stress."

› Positive strategies for managing stress include: exercise, clarifying your worries, and practising the relaxation response.

Chapter Sixteen References

1 Selye, H (1956), *The Stress of Life,* McGraw-Hill.

2 Terre, L (2010), "Is There a Connection Between Diabetes and Psychological Dysfunction?" *American Journal of Lifestyle Medicine,* Vol 4, pages 481-4.

3 American Psychological Association (2010), "Psychologically Healthy Workplace Program: Fact Sheet," <www.apa.org/practice/programs/workplace/phwp-fact-sheet.pdf>.

4 American Psychological Association (2009), "Stress in America 2009 Study" <www.apa.org/news/press/releases/stress-exec-summary.pdf>

5 Williams, J E, et al (2000), "Anger Proneness Predicts Coronary Heart Disease Risk: Prospective Analysis From the Atherosclerosis Risk In Communities (ARIC) Study," *Circulation,* Vol 101 No 17, pages 2034-9.

6 Peters, A, et al (2004), "Exposure to Traffic and the Onset of Myocardial Infarction," *New England Journal of Medicine,* Vol 351 No 17, pages 1721-30.

7 Yusuf, S, et al (2004), "Effect of potentially modifiable risk factors associated with myocardial infarction in 52 countries (the INTERHEART study): case-control study," *Lancet,* Vol 364 No 9438, pages 937-52.

8 Kent, L K, and P A Shapiro (2009), "Depression and Related Psychological Factors in Heart Disease," *Harvard Review of Psychiatry,* Vol 17 No 6, pages 377-88.

9 Beaumont, W (1838), *Experiments and Observations on the Gastric Juice and the Physiology of Digestion,* MacLachlan & Stewart, Edinburgh.

10 Mertz, H (not dated), "Stress and the Gut," University of North Carolina For Functional GI & Motility Disorders, <www.med.unc.edu/ibs/files/educational-gi-handouts/Stress%20and%20the%20Gut.pdf>.

11 Mayer, E (2011), "Gut feelings: the emerging biology of gut-brain communication," *Nature Reviews,* Vol 12, pages 453-66.

12 ibid.

13 Solomon, G F, and R H Moos (1964), "Emotions, immunity, and disease: a speculative theoretical integration," *Archives of General Psychiatry,* Vol 11 No 6, pages 657-74.

14 Kiecolt-Glaser, J K, et al (2002), "Psychoneuroimmunology: Psychological Influences on Immune Function and Health," *Journal of Consulting and Clinical Psychology,* Vol 70 No 3, pages 537-47.

15 Kiecolt-Glaser (2002), ibid.

16 Marucha, P T, et al (1998), "Mucosal wound healing is impaired by examination stress," *Psychosomatic Medicine,* Vol 60, pages 362-365.

17 Kiecolt-Glaser, J K, et al (2005), "Hostile Marital Interactions, Proinflammatory Cytokine Production, and Wound Healing," *Archive of General Psychiatry,* Vol 62 No 12, pages 1377-84.

18 Hart, A (1995), *Adrenaline and Stress: The Exciting New Breakthrough That Helps You Overcome Stress Damage,* Thomas Nelson, pages 31-46.

19 Sapolsky, R M (2004), *Why Zebras Don't Get Ulcers* (Third Edition), Henry Holt and Company.

20 Weil, A, "Foreword" in Rossman, M (2010), *The Worry Solution: Using Breakthrough Brain Science to Turn Stress and Anxiety Into Confidence and Happiness,* Crown Archetype.

21 Benson, H, and W Proctor (2010), *Relaxation Revolution: Enhancing Your Personal Health Through the Science and Genetics of Mind Body Healing,* Scribner.

22 Benson, H, and M Klipper (2000), *The Relaxation Response* (Expanded and Updated Edition), William Morrow Paperbacks.

23 Hart, op cit, page 166.

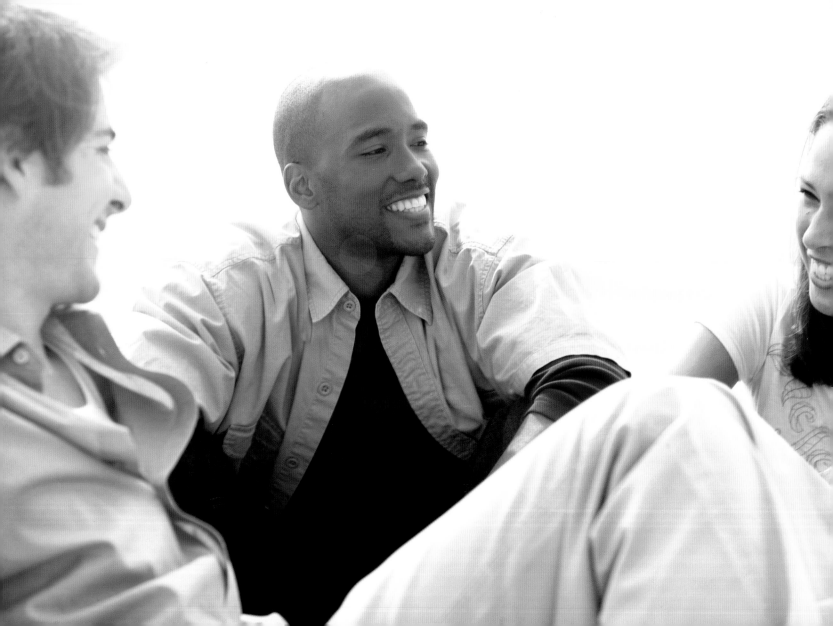

Chapter Seventeen

Fix How You Feel

Many people mistakenly think the quality of our life is determined by things such as wealth, status or career, but these things are merely vehicles to emotions—sometimes good, sometimes bad. Those things that fill us with positive emotions add to our quality of life, whereas those evoking negative emotions detract from our quality of life. It is a worthwhile exercise identifying the things in our life that act as wings and those that are weights.

While the quality of our life is powerfully influenced by our emotional state, so too is the quality of our health. So it makes sense that positive emotions are worth embracing. Unfortunately, an increasing number of people are finding positive emotions difficult to come by. Across the world, rates of depression are skyrocketing and depression is projected to be the second biggest cause of premature death and disability for both males and females of all ages by 2020.[1]

Important note: there is a difference between feeling a "little down" and clinical depression. No-one can expect to consistently feel a 10-out-of-10, day-in day-out, but clinical depression is a medical condition, not unlike a broken arm or diabetes, and for this reason requires expert attention.

However, there is a lot we can do to improve our mood on a daily basis. Let's explore five tips that can help fix how you feel.

While the quality of our life is powerfully influenced by our emotional state, so too is the quality of our health.

Tip 1: **Eat nutritiously**

Throughout this book, we have explained the power of a whole-foods-as-grown eating pattern for improving physical health. However, there is good evidence that eating this way—the diet we were designed for—is not only good for our bodies, it is also great for our minds. Studies have shown that the optimal lifestyle significantly improves participants' mental health by decreasing depression scores.[3] Indeed, many CHIP participants claim that soon after commencing the program they feel like a "fog" lifts, and they can think more clearly and feel better emotionally.

So why can eating a nutritious, plant-based diet improve our mood? Nutrition is a complicated area and various individual nutrients have been suggested to improve mood, such as tryptophan and omega-3 fatty acids.[4] But we all know what it feels like when we've missed a meal. Maybe we have been busy at work or stuck in traffic on our way home, but whatever the reason, it makes us irritable, maybe even lethargic. This is one simple way food directly affects our mood in everyday life.

A more complex example: foods high in processed sugars can cause our blood-sugar levels to skyrocket, which in turn causes our body to produce high levels of insulin. As a result, this actually causes our blood-sugar level to fall below normal levels—a phenomenon referred to as reactive hypoglycemia. Obviously this yo-yo effect on our blood sugar levels does not bode well for our mood and energy levels. Interestingly, the sugars in whole fruits do not tend to wreak the same havoc with our blood-sugar levels.

Similarly, high-fat meals can cause our blood to become "thicker" meaning it doesn't flow as well. From experience, you might identify with how sluggish a high-fat meal can make you feel. Once again, plant-based foods tend to be naturally low in fat, avoiding this problem. Again, when it comes to feeling great, a whole-food plant-based diet comes out on top.

Tip 2: Move dynamically

We have already seen that physical activity can make you feel better by changing your brain chemistry for the better, stimulating the release of feel-good chemicals such as beta endorphins. We have also seen that exercise is a powerful strategy for managing stress by winding down our body's stress response. So moving dynamically has a profound ability to fix how we feel. Researchers have concluded that "young and elderly individuals who engage in programs of exercise display fewer depressive symptoms and are less likely to subsequently develop major depressive disorders."[5]

There is no doubt that what we do with our body affects our mind, thanks in part to many nerve endings distributed throughout our body, called proprioceptors. Proprioceptors are specialized sensory nerve endings found in muscles, tendons and joints that relay information to our brain about our body position and movement in space. When these proprioceptors are dynamically activated, they flood our brain with stimulating messages.

Interestingly, the part of the brain tremendously influenced by proprioceptors is the limbic system, which is responsible for our emotional state. It is our feeling center, so motion creates emotion. But not only is our limbic system responsible for emotions, it is also involved in our motivations and drives.[6] This is why moving dynamically not only makes us feel better, it also makes us feel more motivated.

Consider the example of a warm-up. While warming up before exercise is helpful for increasing our body temperature and limbering up our muscles, it also has the effect of making us feel more like doing the activity to come. Hence, a warm-up prepares us both physiologically and psychologically. If you struggle to find the motivation to go for a 30-minute brisk walk, commit to doing just five minutes, then reassess the situation. Invariably, after five minutes of moving dynamically, you feel ready for another 25 minutes!

When these proprioceptors are dynamically activated, they flood our brain with stimulating messages.

Tip 3: Go natural

There is something incredibly therapeutic about immersing oneself in natural environments, and we seem to know this both consciously and subconsciously. Majestic scenery and landscapes captivate us—even when only presented in two-dimensional photographs. And to find peace and tranquility we gravitate to natural environments such as forests and beaches. Researchers have found a number of links between exposure to nature and elevated health and mood:

- **Nature can make us feel more alive.** Hospital patients who have a view of a natural landscape have shorter hospital stays and tend to consume less painkilling medication.[7]

- **Exposure to nature promotes health-oriented behaviors.** For example, in a study that followed up 1400 individuals several years after they participated in a two-week wilderness course, 90 per cent were able to break unhealthy habits such as the consumption of alcohol and tobacco.[8]

- **Nature can help us feel well by enhancing our relationships.** Researchers have found that spending time in nature can improve social bonds and community ties. Residents of urban housing developments, who frequented treed public spaces, spoke more to other people, were more likely to know their neighbors by name and reported feeling a greater sense of community.[9] Exposure to "green" areas has also been associated with less aggression and even just a window view of nature is significantly correlated to lower levels of domestic violence.[10]

- **"Green" spaces help reduce mental fatigue.** This is explained by the "attention restoration hypothesis," which proposes that natural stimuli including landscapes and animals effortlessly engage our attention. In contrast, modern living makes high demands of our information-processing skills in the form of things such as computers, mobile phones and traffic, which results in unnatural mental strain leading to mental fatigue.[11]

Just a window view of nature is significantly correlated to lower levels of domestic violence.

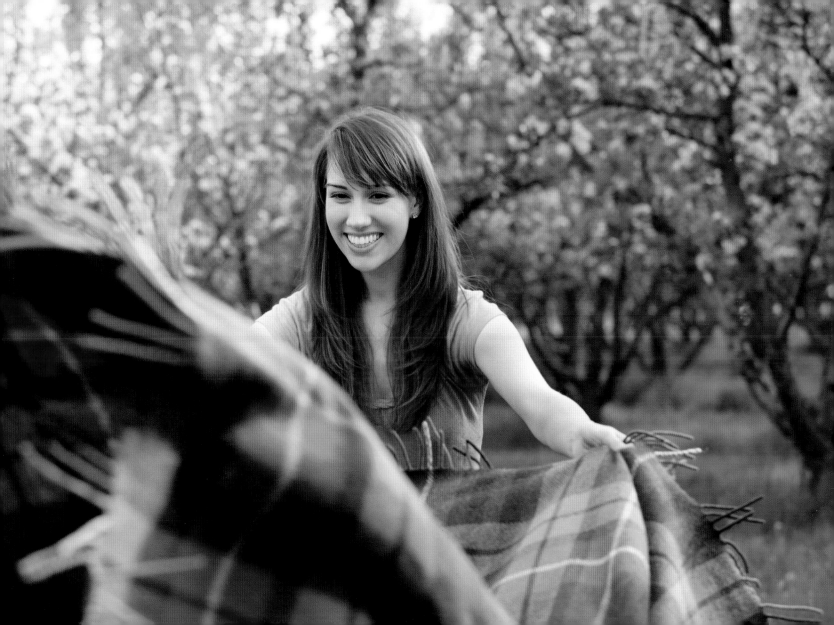

Alarmingly, many people today live in artificial environments and are starved of the natural world we are designed to inhabit. In recognition of this reality, a new term has been coined: "nature deficit disorder." Children suffering nature deficit disorder, who don't get to regularly surround themselves with the great outdoors, are more prone to anxiety, depression, attention deficit disorder and even being overweight.[12]

Two of the most important elements of the natural world that we should be especially mindful of in the pursuit of total wellbeing are fresh air and sunshine.

Fresh air contributes to good health and positive wellbeing as it nurtures almost every cell in our body. Inhaling air contaminated by pollutants can be perilous to our health—smoking being a case in point. Unfortunately, the air space surrounding many cities of the world is polluted. Those who live in such environments should endeavor to escape to the great outdoors as often as able.

Alarmingly, many people today live in an artificial environment and are starved of the natural world we are designed to inhabit.

Sunshine is tremendously important for our wellbeing—in the right doses. While too much sunlight exposure can damage our skin and even cause skin cancers, lack of sunlight can cause low mood and other problems. For example, in regions that get little sunshine during the winter months a condition described as "Seasonal Affective Disorder" is common, and is associated with depression and tragically a high rate of suicide.[13]

Sunlight is also powerfully involved in regulating our "body clock." Sunlight contacting our eyes in the morning helps reset our sleep-wake cycle. Hence, getting some sunshine in the morning is a great way to help fix how we feel, signaling our brains that it is time to wake up and get into the day.

There is something about nature that does us good—we are designed to inhabit it! Make use of the parks, mountains, lakes, forests and beaches you have access to and you will feel better for it.

Tip 4: Rest well

Have you ever been so tired you could hardly keep your eyes open? When we are overcome with weariness, we certainly don't feel full of joy. Just ask Randy Gardner who made it into the *Guinness Book of Records* for going without sleep for 264 hours (or 11 days). After just four days, Randy became delusional, thinking he was someone he wasn't and mistaking road signs for people.

But even only a few nights of inadequate sleep can compromise our wellbeing. One reason lack of sleep is so bad for our wellbeing is because it makes us more clumsy and lacking in good judgment. An Australian study has found that after just 17 hours without sleep, an individual's response speed can be reduced by 50 per cent and their performance can be worse than having a blood alcohol limit of 0.05 per cent.[14] It is not surprising, therefore, that many accounts of major incidents such as oil tankers running aground and planes crashing have been linked to fatigue. Even the devastating *Challenger* space shuttle accident has been traced back to crucial errors of judgment attributed to sleep deprivation.[15]

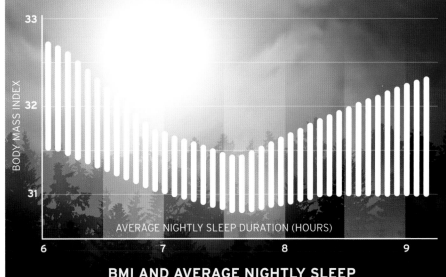

BMI AND AVERAGE NIGHTLY SLEEP

A study of individuals in the Wisconsin Sleep Cohort Study revealed a U-shaped relationship between an individual's average sleep duration and their Body Mass Index. In the study, the individuals who got 7.7 hours of sleep on a typical night had the lowest Body Mass Indexes. Above or below this, Body Mass Index tended to go up, but it was especially pronounced for the short sleepers.[16] The researchers discovered that the short sleepers had significantly higher levels of the hormone ghrelin, and lower levels of leptin in their bodies. Ghrelin is the hormone that makes us feel hungry, whereas leptin make us feel satiated. Hence, when we are tired we are more inclined to eat more.[17]

But aside from accidents, lack of sleep is related to increased risks of type 2 diabetes, cardiovascular disease and premature death from all causes,[18] and contributes to obesity.[19]

While lack of sleep contributes to obesity, obesity can also contribute to poorer sleep. When you put on weight in your neck area, it thickens not just outward but also inward, and the inward thickening can cause your windpipe to close when the muscles around it relax during sleep. This is referred to as obstructive sleep apnea. It is extremely common and terribly disruptive to sleep. While we might not even be aware of constantly being woken, sleep apnea devastates our sleep quality and is one of the leading causes of day-time sleepiness. If you suspect you could be a sufferer, talk with your health professional. It can make a huge difference to your quality of life.

Sleep also has a huge effect on our brains.[20] It is important for memory as it is needed for the development of new brain cells and forging connections between them.[21] Studies show that people who are taught a mentally challenging task do better after a good night's sleep, and research suggests that sleep is needed for creative problem solving. Further, lack of sleep is associated with anxiety disorders and depression.[22]

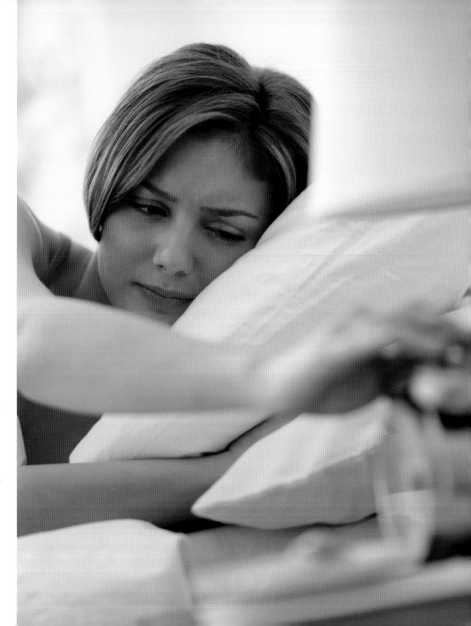

How to improve the quality of your sleep

Tips from the National Institutes of Health:[23]

> ### › Stick to a sleep schedule.

Go to bed and wake up at much the same time each day if you can—even on weekends. Within our brain is a small bundle of cells that control our "body clock," which determines natural cycles ("circadian rhythms") that occur over a 24-hour period in which we feel awake and alert, then sleepy. Keeping a regular sleep-wake cycle allows our body clock to synchronize, so we are more inclined to feel awake when we are meant to and sleepy when it is time to go to bed.

> ### › Be active in the morning light.

One of the best ways to reset your body clock is to expose yourself to sunshine when you wake up in the morning. When sunlight hits your eyes, your body clock decreases the production of the sleep hormone melatonin. While you are out in the sun, do something active as exercise is also well known to help with sleep. However, it is best to exercise at least two hours before you are planning to sleep if you find it hypes you up.

> ### › Avoid things that keep you up.

Television and computers are distractions that commonly eat into sleep time. However, eating and drinking too late can also keep us awake as they can disturb our sleep quality. Of course, caffeinated products are particularly problematic because the stimulating effects of caffeine can take up to eight hours to fully wear off!

Contrary to popular thought, alcoholic drinks are not helpful for getting good sleep. While a "nightcap" might help you fall asleep, the alcohol keeps you in the lighter stages of sleep so the sleep is not as good quality. Also you tend to wake up in the middle of the night when the sedating effects wear off.

While day time naps can be rejuvenating, keep them early in the day—definitely before 3 pm—and don't let them extend for more than an hour, otherwise they can interrupt your sleep that night.

> ### › Get relaxed and comfortable.

Your bed should be the most comfortable place on earth—after all, you spend about one-third of your life in it! Be sure to make it just that. And before you get into it, take time to relax, whether by reading a book, listening to music or having a bath.

Sleep is so important for your health and wellbeing that you can't afford not to make it a priority. If you struggle to get enough quality sleep, take measures to remedy it. If the strategies above are not helpful, talk with your healthcare provider.

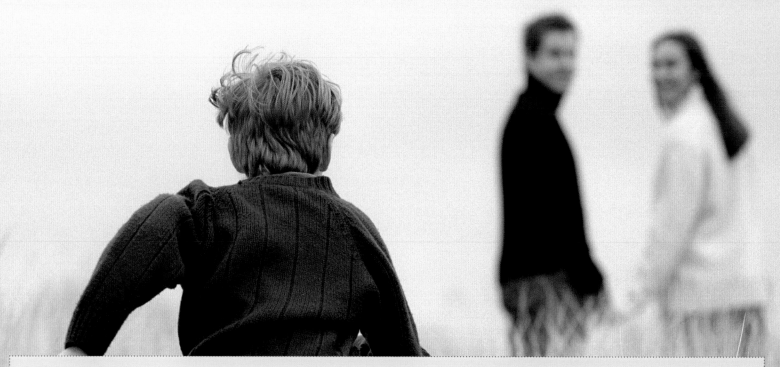

TAKE A DAY OFF

Sleep is only one part of "resting well." So many people today are living at a frantic pace seven days a week. In the 1960s, economists forecasted that our technological breakthroughs would allow us to work only a few hours a week and that our main problem would be deciding what to do with all our leisure time.[24] Of course, nothing could be further from reality for most of us. We are working longer and longer hours, and it is taking its toll on us and our families.

An incredibly powerful strategy for achieving work-life balance and resting well is the principle of "Sabbath." This ancient wisdom can be found in a number of faith traditions. The idea is to take one day each week off from work to nurture the truly important things in life—health, relationships and spirituality. Individuals who incorporate this principle into their lives testify to its healing, rejuvenating and enriching qualities.

Tip 5: Look to the positive

Neuroanatomists have discovered that there is an intimate relationship between our thinking brain—the frontal cortex—and our emotional brain—the limbic system.[25] This means what we think about is what we feel. If you give your attention to and talk about the high things in life—the best and the praiseworthy—it can transform how you feel. And it is possible to develop the skill of being more positive by practising gratitude and optimism.[26]

Ask yourself:

> ### › What in my life am I truly thankful for?

When you give your attention to this question, your emotional brain gets bombarded with positive messages from your frontal cortex and it improves how you feel. In his book, *Authentic Happiness*, researcher and former president of the American Psychological Association, Dr Martin Seligman, says that expressing gratitude is one of the most powerful ways for improving our mood.[27]

> ### › What in my life am I truly excited about?

If you can't name at least one thing you are looking forward to or are truly excited about, you need to do something about it. When we don't have a spirit of anticipation, life becomes dull, boring and mundane. This is one reason children are usually happy and upbeat—they have an innate capacity to get excited. Reflecting on things we are excited about floods our emotional brain with positive messages and can improve our mood.

> ### › What can I do to make someone else feel good?

There seems to be a law that governs how we feel: we reap what we sow. When we intentionally set about dragging others down, we go down with them. But if we purposefully set about raising others up emotionally, we go up with them. Dr Seligman says that after all his research in the field of what makes people happy, one of the take-away messages is "Do something to make someone else happy!"[28]

Emotionally, we reap what we sow. This gives us a powerful strategy for helping to fix how we feel, and an incredible perspective for approaching a life worth living.

KEY POINTS

> The quality of our life is largely determined by the quality of our emotions—how we feel on a consistent basis.

> Strategies to help "fix how you feel" include:

1. Eat nutritiously.

2. Move dynamically.

3. Immerse yourself regularly in the natural world, particularly enjoying fresh air and sunshine.

4. Rest well—sleep enough and take a day off each week.

5. Look to the positive. Be grateful and get excited. Think about others and engage in service activities.

Chapter Seventeen References

1. World Health Organization (2012), "Depression," <http://www.who.int/mental_health/management/depression/definition/en/>.

2. Dunn, E W, et al (2008), "Spending Money on Others Promotes Happiness," *Science*, Vol 319 No 5870, pages 1687-8.

3. Thieszen, C, et al (2011), "The Coronary Health Improvement Project (CHIP) for lowering weight and improving psychosocial health," *Psychological Reports*, Vol 109 No 1, pages 338-52.

4. Nedley, N (2005), *Depression: The Way Out*, Neil Nedley Publishing.

5. Ernst, C, et al (2006), "Antidepressant effects of exercise: Evidence for an adult-neurogenesis hypothesis?" *Journal of Psychiatry and Neuroscience*, Vol 31 No 2, pages 84-92.

6. Clark, D L, et al (2010), *The Brain and Behaviour*, Cambridge University Press.

7. Ulrich, R S (1984), "View Through a Window May Influence Recovery from Surgery," *Science*, Vol 224, pages 420-1.

8. Greenway, R (1995), "The Wilderness Effect and Ecopsychology," in T Roszak, M E Gomes, and A D Kanner (editors), *Ecopsychology: Restoring the earth, healing the mind*, Sierra Book Club.

9. Kuo, F E (2001), "Coping with poverty: Impacts of environment and attention in the inner city," *Environment and Behavior*, Vol 33 No 1, pages 5-34.

10. Kuo, F E, and W C Sullivan (2001), "Aggression and violence in the inner city: Effects of environment via mental fatigue," *Environmental Behavior*, Vol 33 No 4, pages 543-71.

11. Kaplan, S (1995), "The restorative benefits of nature: Toward an integrative framework," *Journal of Environmental Psychiatry*, Vol 15 No 3, pages 169-82.

12. Louv, R (2011), *The Nature Principle: Human restoration and the end of nature-deficit disorder*, Algonquin Books.

13. National Institutes of Health (2011), "Seasonal Affective Disorder," Publication No. 11-5800, <http://www.ncbi.nlm.nih.gov/pubmedhealth/PMH0002499/>.

14. Williamson, A, and A Feyer A (2000), "Moderate sleep deprivation produces impairments in cognitive and motor performance equivalent to legally prescribed levels of alcohol intoxication," *Occupational and Environmental Medicine*, Vol 57, pages 649-55.

15. National Sleep Foundation, <www.sleepfoundation.org>.

16. Taheri, S, et al (2004), "Short sleep duration is associated with reduced leptin, elevated ghrelin, and increased body mass index," *PLoS Medicine*, Vol 1 No 3, page e62.

17. Benedict, C, et al (2012), "Acute Sleep Deprivation Enhances the Brain's Response to Hedonic Food Stimuli: An fMRI Study," *Journal of Clinical Endocrinology and Metabolism*, Vol 97 No 3, page e443.

18. Chien, K L, et al (2010), "Habitual sleep duration and insomnia and the risk of cardio-vascular events and all-cause death: report from a community-based cohort," *Sleep*, Vol 33, pages 177-84; Gallicchio, L,

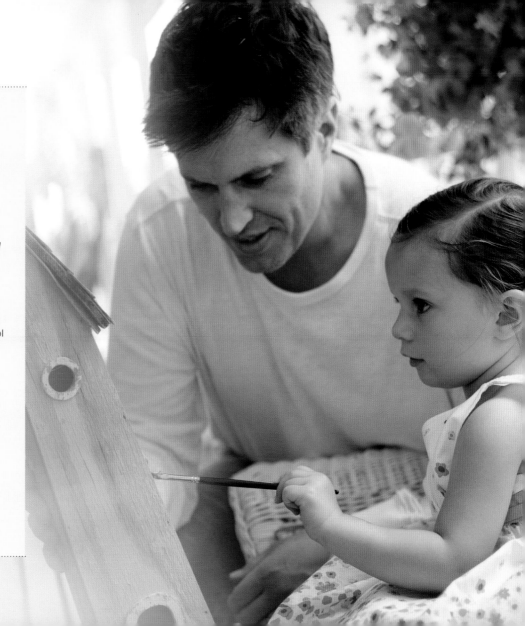

and B Kalesan (2009), "Sleep duration and mortality: a systematic review and meta-analysis," *Journal of Sleep Research,* Vol 18, pages 148-58; Harvard Medical School, Division of Sleep Medicine, <http://healthysleep.med.harvard.edu/healthy/>.

19 Morselli, L, et al (2012), "Sleep and metabolic function," *European Journal of Physiology,* Vol 463 No 1, pages 139-60.

20 Banks, S, and D F Dinges (2007), "Behavioral and physiological consequences of sleep restriction," *Journal of Clinical Sleep Medicine,* Vol 3 No 5, pages 519-28.

21 Meerlo, P, et al (2009), "New neurons in the adult brain: The role of sleep and consequences of sleep loss," *Sleep Medicine Reviews,* Vol 13 No 3, pages 187-94.

22 Neckelmann, D, et al (2007), 'Chronic Insomnia As a Risk Factor for Developing Anxiety and Depression," *Sleep,* Vol 30 No 7, pages 873-80.

23 National Institutes of Health (2012), "Your guide to healthy sleep," <www.nhlbi.nih.gov/sleep>.

24 Hamilton, C, and R Denniss (2006), *Affluenza: When too much is never enough,* Allen & Unwin.

25 Clark, op cit.

26 Lyubomirsky, S, et al (2011), "Becoming Happier Takes Both a Will and a Proper Way: An experimental longitudinal intervention to boost well-being," *Emotion,* Vol 11 No 2, pages 391-402.

27 Seligman, M (2002), *Authentic Happiness,* Free Press.

28 Seligman, M (2004), TED talk, <www.ted.com/talks/lang/en/martin_seligman_on_the_state_of_psychology.html>.

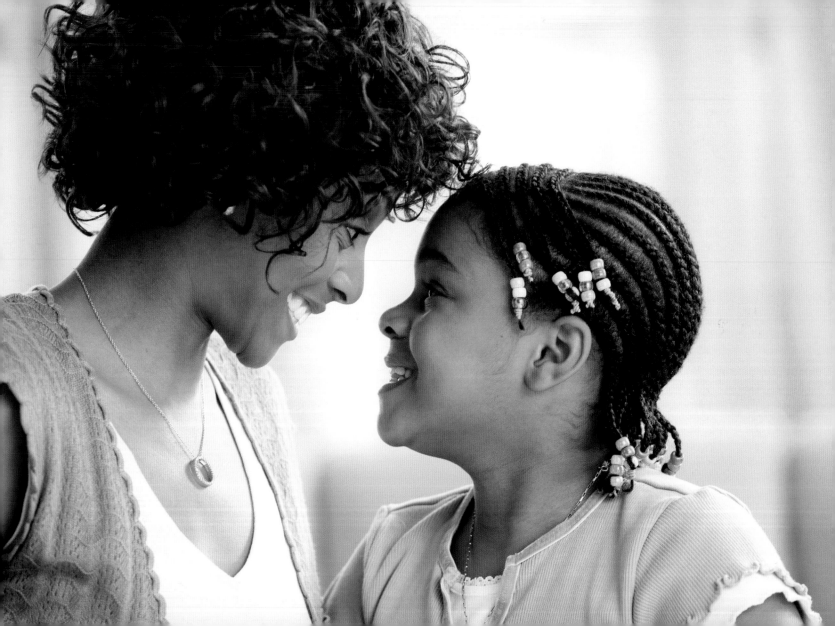

Chapter Eighteen

From Surviving to Thriving

In 1997, Dr Martin Seligman was voted as president of the American Psychological Association and he decided to invest his energies and influence into a new field of psychology. Dr Seligman noted that psychology had concerned itself traditionally only with the negative–devoting all its attention to remedying dysfunctional psychological states–so he decided to investigate and promote what he referred to as *positive psychology*.[1] Positive psychology does not refer to the idea of "thinking yourself happy" or wishful thinking, rather the intent of positive psychology is to scientifically understand and promote thriving individuals, families and communities in order to make "normal" lives more fulfilling.[2] A key concept in the field is that true happiness has a number of important contributing factors. Just as in whole-person health, these factors can be valuable on their own, but it's when all factors come together like a jigsaw puzzle that the biggest impact on wellbeing is felt.

Initially, positive psychology literature focused on *happiness*–what causes it, how to achieve it, and its associated benefits. These studies noted that happy people tend to be healthier and even live longer. For example, nuns who penned more optimistic, "happier" life sketches when entering the convent lived longer than their more pessimistic friends. Similarly, the longevity of major league baseball players was correlated to the extent to which they smiled on their baseball card photo.[3]

However, while happiness is a worthy pursuit, it takes more than just smiles and giggles to thrive in life. More recently, Dr Seligman has suggested that the higher ideal is to *flourish*. Flourishing is a more comprehensive measure of what it takes to live well and it encapsulates five domains, with the later ones supplying the deeper levels of life satisfaction and fulfillment.

Let's consider what it takes to live a life that flourishes.

The higher ideal is to flourish. Flourishing is a more comprehensive measure of what it takes to live well.

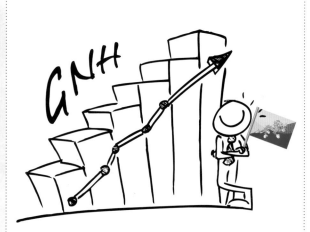

A DIFFERENT MEASURE

Recognizing the merits of happiness, some countries like Bhutan have begun thinking differently about how the success of a nation should be measured, adopting Gross National Happiness (GNH) as the guiding philosophy behind its development rather than the conventional Gross Domestic Product (GDP).[4] After all, GDP is not necessarily a good measure of the wellbeing of a nation as it increases with "each sale of antidepressant medication, with each divorce pronounced, and with each prison built."[5]

1. Positive emotions

A life filled with positive emotions—such as joy, happiness, peace, contentment, excitement and ecstasy—makes for a "pleasant life". Not surprisingly, people who have more positive emotion are more satisfied with their lives.[6]

But not only is a life filled with positive emotions more satisfying, it is also likely to be longer. One reason for this is that positive emotion has been shown to trigger a range of health-promoting benefits, as we have seen. The consensus of numerous studies conducted on just one of the many positive emotions—humor—indicate that the ancient proverb was right when it asserted, "A cheerful heart is good like medicine."[7] Humor and laughter strengthen the immune system, reduce pain, lower blood pressure (over time), relax muscles and reduce blood levels of stress-related hormones.[8]

It is good to enjoy positive emotions as often as we are able but positive emotions are not always easy to come by. We all experience events in our lives that cause happy feelings to evaporate and it is appropriate to experience negative emotions at such times. It is unrealistic to think we can live in a state of perpetual bliss. And even in the absence of crises, being cheery is more difficult for some than others. It is estimated that genetics contributes about 50 per cent to our ability to harness positive emotions.[9]

There are other reasons why a life dedicated to the pursuit of pleasure is problematic:

› **Positive emotions don't last.** While pleasure should be savored when it comes into our lives, laughter is never limitless and pleasure is never permanent. Even the best joke loses its impact the fourth time around.

› **When positive emotions are over, they are over.** An episode of uncontrollable laughter will not satisfy us for weeks or even days. To "flourish" through the pursuit of pleasure, we will need to constantly busy ourselves seeking it. As John D Rockefeller once said, "I can think of nothing less pleasurable than a life devoted to pleasure."

This is not to deride the enjoyment or benefits of positive emotion as an important ingredient of a flourishing life. But as Dr Seligman and other researchers have discovered, it should not be our highest pursuit.

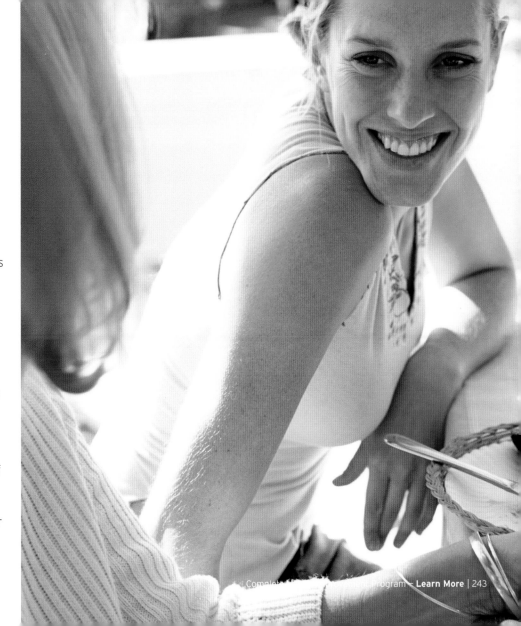

2. Engagement

Have you ever been so completely engrossed in a particular activity that when you looked up some time later you were surprised by how much time had passed?

A pioneering researcher in the field of positive psychology, Dr Mihaly Csikszentmihalyi has studied intensively this experience he describes as "flow"—a state of heightened focus and immersion that occurs in activities such as art, play and work. Not surprisingly, individuals who report high levels of flow in their daily activities, leading to *engagement,* report higher levels of life satisfaction—and are more inclined to flourish.

Because we spend so much of our time working, it is ideal to find employment that engages us. But it is not what you do that matters, it is what it *means* to you. Regardless of the area of employment, those who are most engaged are those who view what they do not as just a *job* or even a *career,* but a *calling.* Typically, we are more likely to feel called to a task when we are able to apply our unique strengths and talents to it.

Sadly, Gallup researchers found that only about 20 per cent of individuals report a strong "yes" to the question "Do you like what you do each day?"[10] And they found those who were less engaged in their work had higher levels of the stress hormone cortisol. But even if you don't wake up excited on workdays, having something to do each day appears imperative for our wellbeing. Researchers from the Centre of Economic Performance found that sustained unemployment can be incredibly damaging to our wellbeing, even more than the death of a spouse. In their study, four years after losing a spouse, men's wellbeing scores had mostly recovered whereas their wellbeing scores still suffered four years after a prolonged period of unemployment.[11]

If we are not engaged in our work, it is even more critical that we engage in regular play. By definition, play refers to activities we do for the sheer enjoyment of them—no extrinsic reward required. As adults, we tend to lose the capacity to play, which does us a great disservice. Interestingly, engaging in play is considered a sign of intelligence in the animal kingdom—monkeys play, dogs play, dolphins play but amoebas don't. So it is ironic that while children are the play masters, adults seem to lose the ability. We need to reclaim it!

3. Accomplishment

If you are a person who judges whether a day has been good or bad according to how many items on your "to do" list you were able to tick off, you will agree that there is something rewarding about achieving something that you have set your mind to. Unfortunately, if you are that kind of person, you probably also have a tendency to overestimate what you are capable of achieving in any given day, so invariably feel dissatisfied with how few of the items on your list you crossed off!

Dr Seligman suggests that a sense of achievement, accomplishment, success or mastery can help people flourish. Accomplishment can be achieved in many domains, including sports, business or education. Sometimes it is measured through agreed standards such as competitions, awards or performing at a particular level. At an individual level, accomplishment can be defined in terms of feelings, lifestyles and attaining goals.

Accomplishment can enrich our lives independently of positive emotion or engagement. There are many tasks that don't fill us with joyful emotions at the time of performing them or captivate our attention, yet on their completion we discover a deep satisfaction that motivates us to do it again. For example, athletes often talk about how painful an event was and how the last stage of the race felt like it would never end but then start planning how they can do it again.

The accomplishment of worthwhile pursuits can add value to our lives. However, accomplishment does not represent the highest ideals in the quest to flourish. In fact, a life dedicated in an unbalanced way to accomplishment can compromise the next, more important, component of a well-lived life.

Accomplishment can enrich our lives independently of positive emotion or engagement.

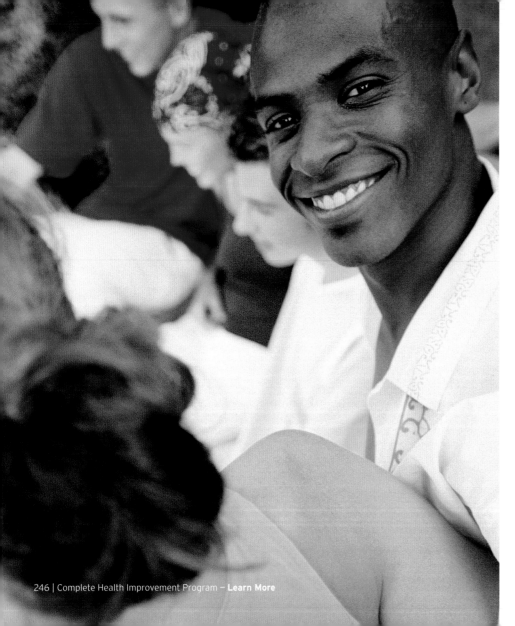

4. Relationships

Human beings are relational creatures and our deepest levels of wellbeing seem to be realized by loving and being loved: "The belief that one is cared for, loved, esteemed, and valued has been recognized as one of the most (if not the most) influential determinants of wellbeing for people of all ages and cultures."[12] When researchers study the top 10 per cent of happy people, the single most important factor that emerges is that these very happy people have good social relationships.[13] We seek connectedness—and that connectedness helps us flourish.

Studies show that our relationships and support networks can have a tremendous influence on our quality of life, health and longevity. One of the world's leading experts in the field of lifestyle medicine, Dr Dean Ornish, comments, "Anything that promotes a sense of isolation often leads to illness and suffering. Anything that promotes a sense of love and intimacy, connection and community, is healing."[14] Numerous studies show that positive, supportive relationships boost immune function, while negative relationships impair immune function. These findings are so consistent that experts in the field have concluded, "The link between personal relationships and immune function is one of the most robust findings in psychoneuroimmunology."[15] It is little wonder that in Dan Buettner's study of the "Blue Zones"—pockets on the globe where individuals live extraordinarily long lives—a high level of social support was a common theme.[16]

Although the extent to which this occurs is only just being recognized, our relationships also have a tremendous influence on our level of happiness. A recent study by Harvard researchers found that happy people can infectiously spread their joy up to three degrees of separation—which means the friends of their friends receive a mood lift![17] From personal experience, we know that some people are uplifting to be around, while others are less so. As Oscar Wilde once commented, "Some people bring happiness *wherever* they go, others bring happiness *whenever* they go!"

It helps to seek out positive influences or—better still—be one. However, not all relationships are positive. While positive relationships can enrich our lives, negative relationships can reduce us to lows we probably would not reach on our own. Relationships can magnify emotions. They can cause good times to reach higher peaks but the lows can sink to deeper depths.

In the pursuit of our best life, positive relationships and social support are absolutely necessary. We should actively seek to strengthen our existing relationships and create new ones, if needed. There are great benefits associated with finding uplifting friends, and a great place to start is by joining positive groups, such as sporting clubs and church groups. Strengthening our current connections can be greatly assisted through prioritization. "Spending time" is integral to the formation of robust relationships and building understanding even in sometimes-difficult relationships.

Relationships can magnify emotions. They can cause good times to reach higher peaks but the lows can sink to deeper depths.

5. Meaning

We can have a life bursting with fun times, be engaged in our daily activities, achieve significant things and feel connected to others, yet—in our quieter moments—we can still find ourselves wondering about the point of it all. Having a sense of *meaning* is a fundamental need of humans. It is difficult—perhaps impossible—to live a flourishing life without it.

Dr Seligman defines meaning as a feeling of "belonging to and serving something that you believe is bigger than the self."[18] Tragically, we live in an increasingly egocentric society, appropriately described as the "I" generation. Yet, there is overwhelming evidence that the best thing we can do to thrive is to purposefully look outside ourselves and beyond our own interests to help others thrive. At an emotional level, we reap what we sow. And acts of service reap more than just warm fuzzy feelings; we gain a greater sense that our life has meaning.

We also discover meaning in our life when we gain a sense of our true identity. CHIP comes from a philosophy that believes every person is significant and immeasurably valuable. You are of incredible worth. Allowing that truth to sink into the depths of your psyche will transform your sense of meaning. But at CHIP we also believe that every person has been created with a unique set of talents and abilities. Armed with the knowledge that you matter, you will discover a deep level of meaning when you activate your unique set of strengths for the service of others.

Here is your challenge: "Make a careful exploration of who you are and the work you have been given, and then sink yourself into it. Don't be impressed with yourself. Don't compare yourself with others. Each of you must take responsibility for doing the creative best you can with your own life."[19] Only when we recognize that our strengths and skills are for service, not status, do we truly come alive.

When we approach life from this perspective the entire "Flourish" equation balances. We are flooded with positive emotions, we are highly engaged, our achievements are rewarding beyond compare and we discover a deep level of connection. And that connection occurs not only with other people. We also begin to sense a connection with something bigger than ourselves that speaks meaning into our lives in a profound way. That reality can make our life truly flourish.

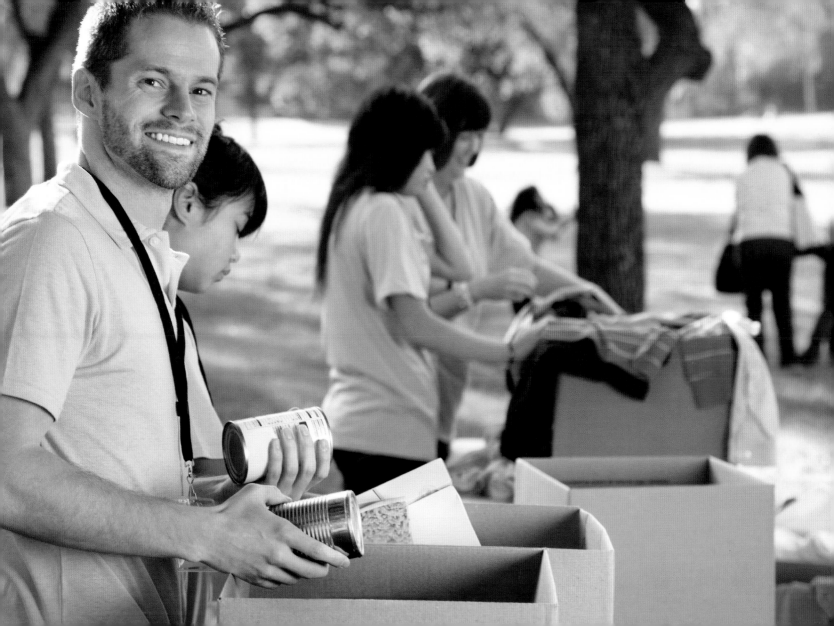

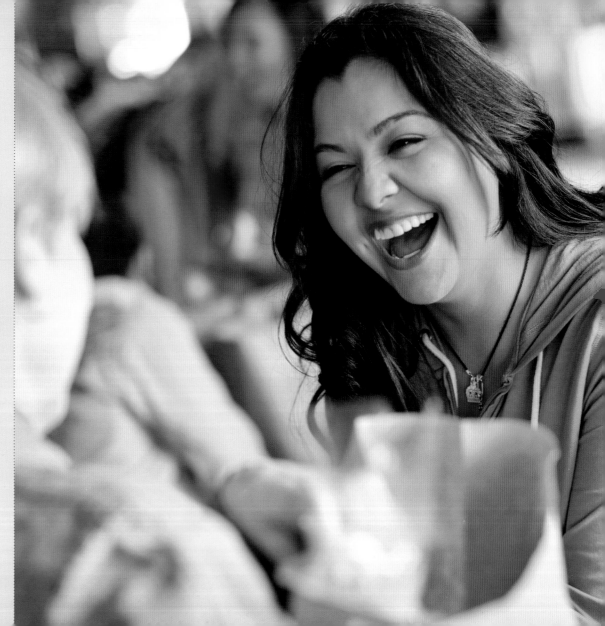

KEY POINTS

› Since the late 1990s, researchers in positive psychology have endeavored to understand and promote thriving individuals, families and communities.

› Pursuit of pleasure does not bring true happiness. We should enjoy moments of pleasure in our lives, but to achieve true happiness, they should not be our highest pursuit.

› Research in positive psychology has identified that in order to "flourish," people need to tend to five domains (in order of increasing importance):
  • positive emotion
  • engagement
  • achievement
  • positive relationships, and
  • meaning.

Chapter Eighteen References

1 Seligman, M (2002), *Authentic Happiness: Using the New Positive Psychology to Realize Your Potential for Lasting Fulfillment*, Free Press, pages 28-9.

2 Seligman, M, and M Csikszentmihalyi (2000), "Positive Psychology: An Introduction," *American Psychologist*, Vol 55 No 1, pages 5-14.

3 Seligman, M (2011), *Flourish: A Visionary New Understanding of Happiness and Well-being*, Simon & Schuster, page 221.

4 Thinley, J (2010), "What is Gross National Happiness?" in R McDonald, *Taking Happiness Seriously: Eleven Dialogues on Gross National Happiness*, Centre for Bhutan Studies, pages 1-11.

5 Forgeard, M, et al (2011), "Doing the right thing: Measuring wellbeing for public policy," *International Journal of Wellbeing*, Vol 1 No 1, pages 79-106.

6 Diener, E, and R Biswas-Diener (2008), *Happiness: Unlocking the mysteries of psychological wealth*, Wiley-Blackwell, pages 30, 139.

7 Bible, Proverbs 17:22.

8 McGhee, P (2010), *Humor: The lighter path to resilience and health*, Author House.

9 Seligman (2002), op cit, page 47.

10 Rath, T, and J Harter (2010), *Wellbeing: The five essential elements*, Gallup Press, page 15.

11 Clark, A, et al (2008), "Lags And Leads in Life Satisfaction: a Test of the Baseline Hypothesis," *The Economic Journal*, Vol 118 No 529, pages F222-43.

12 Reis, H, and S Gable (2003), "Toward a positive psychology of relationships" in C Keyes and J Haidt (editors), *Flourishing: Positive psychology and the life well-lived*, American Psychological Association.

13 Seligman (2002), op cit.

14 Ornish, D (1999), *Love and Survival: 8 Pathways to Intimacy and Health*, HarperCollins, page 14.

15 Kiecolt-Glaser, J K, et al (2002), "Psychoneuroimmunology: Psychological Influences on Immune Function and Health," *Journal of Consulting and Clinical Psychology*, Vol 70 No 3, pages 537-47.

16 Buettner, D (2008), *The Blue Zones: Lessons for living longer from the people who have lived the longest*, National Geographic Society, pages 256-8.

17 Fowler, J H, and N A Christakis (2008), "Dynamic spread of happiness in a large social network: longitudinal analysis over 20 years in the Framingham Heart Study," *British Medical Journal*, Vol 337, page a2338.

18 Seligman (2011), op cit, page 17.

19 *The Message*, Galatians 6.

Index

effect on DNA, 187

for heart disease, 41

for optimal health, 19-29

liver cancer, 114

lymphatic system, 106

M

macular degeneration, 36, 41

meat

as iron source, 128

as protein source, 124

consumption, 57, 112

medicine: models of

allopathic medicine, 9

differences between conventional and lifestyle medicine, 27

historical view, 8

lifestyle medicine, 20

patient-centered care, 28

Morris, Dr Jerry, 136

N

National Health Survey, 84

National Heart, Lung, and Blood Institute, 20

nitric oxide, 37

nuts, 57

calcium in almonds, 122

fiber content, 67

iron content, 128

protein in almonds, 126

O

obesity

and aerobic exercises, 152

and emotional distress, 217

and your environment, 197-206

gene connection, 190

link to breast cancer survival, 108

link to disease development, 24, 34, 95

link to energy-dense food, 110

link to inactivity, 136, 143

reducing risks of, 127

relationship to sleep, 234

socially contagious, 203

trends in America, 196

O'Dea, Dr Karen, 98

Okinawans, 138

Ornish, Dr Dean, 24, 112, 246

osteoblast, 119, 120

osteoclast, 119, 120

osteoporosis, 120, 131, 140

oxidative stress

common causes, 41

definition, 35

reduce amount, 81-82

P

pasta

fiber content, 66

penicillin, 8

peripheral neuropathy

link to poor circulation, 36

physical activity, 138-140

see also exercise

positive psychology, 241, 244

potassium, 86

prebiotics, 65

pregnancy

and diabetes, 95

and vitamin B12, 130

cause of constipation, 69

diet connection to future generations, 190

recommended iron intake, 128

probiotics, 65

yoghurt, 65

protein, 50

requirements, 122, 124

sources of, 55, 124-126

protein requirements, 124

R

reactive hypoglycemia, 228

recreation, 137

red meat

see meat

red wine, 113

relationships, 246

relaxation

reversing stress, 223

research studies

Adventist Health Study 2, 22-23

China Study, 21

EPIC Norfolk Study, 21

Framingham Heart Study, 20

resistant starch, 64

Rockefeller, John D, 243

S

sabbath, 236

salt, *see* sodium

Sapolsky, Robert, 220

sarcopenia, 154

Sardinians, 138

saturated fat, 81, 120-121

seasonal affective disorder, 232

Seligman, Dr Martin, 237, 241, 243, 245, 248

Selye, Dr Hans, 211-212

Serenity Prayer, 222

Seventh-day Adventists, 22-23, 138

skin cancer
  and vitamin D, 123

sleep
  health benefits of, 233-235
  relationship to BMI, 233

smoking
  and bone health, 122
  cardiovascular disease risk factor, 14, 21
  cause of inflammation, 34

social environment, 203

sodium
  content in food, 89-91
  effects on health, 85
  in processed foods, 87
  reduction of, 87

soy products
  and breast cancer, 111
  as source of calcium, 122
  as source of soluble fiber, 64
  goodness of, 111
  high in protein, 55
  iron content, 128
  soy isoflavones, 111
  soy milk and vitamin B12, 57, 130

Stamler, Dr Jeremiah, 38

St Martin, Alexis, 214

stomach cancer, 114

stress, 211-224
  see also distress
  stress-relieving strategies, 217-222

sugar
  as energy source, 50
  content in fruit juice, 110
  from carbohydrates, 55
  how it gets into the blood, 97
  in diet, 98
  in refined and processed food, 56
  promoting weight gain, 110

T

trans fats, 81

transportation, 136

triglycerides, 14, 82

U

University of Arizona Medical School, 222

V

vegetables
  fiber content, 67

vegetarianism
  effects on cholesterol, 24-25
  health benefits, 22-23, 100, 127

iron deficiency, 129

vitamin B12, 130

vitamins
  vitamin B12, 57, 116, 130
  vitamin C, 129
  vitamin D, 80, 123
  danger of skin cancer, 123

W

weight issues, 13-14
  see also obesity
  body fatness, 107

Weil, Dr Andrew, 222

World Cancer Research Fund, 105, 143

World Health Organization (WHO), 19, 79, 106, 121, 124, 200

Y

yoghurt
  source of probiotics, 65